Living Beyond Multiple Sclerosis

Praise for the authors' previous book, *Women Living with Multiple Sclerosis*:

"Nichols and company are particularly helpful in dealing with the uncertainty surrounding diagnosis (MS is notoriously hard to pin down) and the resulting emotional roller coaster. Nichols and her friends have stood up under the trials MS has hurled their way. Their strength and their practical outlook can help others cope."
— Kirkus Reviews

Online reviews and comments from readers:

"I wanted to laugh and cry as I read this book.... I had a hard time putting it down to even eat!" (Illinois)

"A 'must-have' book for anyone living with Multiple Sclerosis.... I hope that there is a Part Two in the works." (Pennsylvania)

"[The members of the group] discuss openly what MS is all about and do it with clarity, but more importantly with a sense of humor and spiritualism." (Idaho)

"This book deals with day to day life problems, with the main point being LIVING!" (Wisconsin)

"The stories the women in this book told could have been told by me. It's very comforting to know that I am not alone." (California)

"ABSOLUTELY PERFECT — read it in two days, felt like I was a part. I reread parts of it often just to feel the support and understanding that is palpable in the pages." (North Carolina)

"More than OUTSTANDING! I am newly diagnosed with MS (only four months). This book was just the thing I needed." (42-year-old mother of three)

"It's a real 'must-read' for anyone close to a woman diagnosed with MS." (38-year-old retired nurse)

"I truly feel that no other book comes close to 'hitting the nail on the head' when it comes to how 'we' feel, both physically and mentally. Get the book, it's worth it." (33-year-old mother of three)

"An informative, well-written, and entertaining book about this dreaded disease. I look forward to another. Write on!!!" (preschool teacher)

Women Living with Multiple Sclerosis won the 1999 *American Journal of Nursing* Book of the Year Award for most outstanding in Consumer Health

---

Ordering

Trade bookstores in the U.S. and Canada, please contact:

Publishers Group West
1700 Fourth Street, Berkeley CA 94710
Phone: (800) 788-3123 Fax: (510) 528-3444

Hunter House books are available at bulk discounts for textbook course adoptions; to qualifying community, health care, and government organizations; and for special promotions and fund-raising. For details please contact:

Special Sales Department
Hunter House Inc., PO Box 2914, Alameda CA 94501-0914
Phone: (510) 865-5282   Fax: (510) 865-4295
E-mail: ordering@hunterhouse.com

Individuals can order our books from most bookstores
or by calling toll-free:
(800) 266-5592

LIVING
BEYOND
MULTIPLE
SCLEROSIS
A Women's Guide

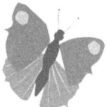

Judith Lynn Nichols
and Her Online Group of MS Sisters

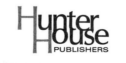

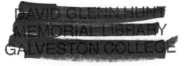

Library of Congress Cataloging-in-Publication Data
Nichols, Judith Lynn.
Living beyond multiple sclerosis: a women's guide / Judith Lynn Nichols.
p. cm.
Includes index.
ISBN 0-89793-293-5 (pbk.)
1. Multiple sclerosis—Popular works. 2. Women—Diseases. I. Title.
RC377 .N527 2000
362.1'96834—dc21

Project Credits
Cover Design: Design Works / Peri Poloni
Book Design and Production: *osprey*design
Developmental Editor: Lydia Bird
Copy Editor: Shila-Vi Alcantara
Proofreader: John David Marion
Indexer: ALTA Indexing
Production Manager: Keri Northcott
Graphics Coordinator: Ariel Parker
Acquisitions Editor: Jeanne Brondino
Associate Editor: Alexandra Mummery
Editorial Intern: Martha Benco
Publicity Manager: Sarah Frederick
Marketing Assistant: Earlita Chenault
Customer Service Manager: Christina Sverdrup
Order Fulfillment: Joel Irons
Publisher: Kiran S. Rana

Printed and Bound by Publishers Press, Salt Lake City, Utah
Manufactured in the United States of America

9 8 7 6 5 4 3 2 1   First Edition   00 01 02 03 04

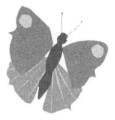

Contents

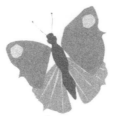

Acknowledgments

I could fill another book with the names of the people who helped me to write this one. Thanks to all of my friends and family who offered support, advice, encouragement, and patience.

Special thanks:

To Kiran Rana and everybody at Hunter House. Once again, our collaboration has been business and pleasure in equal measure;

To the Buds, Flutterers and Gutterers, for going even higher with me;

To Ron, my enabler, my partner, and the love of my life;

To Karen and Julie, my reasons for trying. Your pride makes me proud;

To Bishop Caesar, for the million life-lessons, especially the one about mission;

To Donna Sue, for hanging with me for a lifetime;

To my God, for speaking so clearly once again.

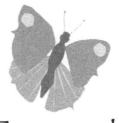

Foreword

A patient walks into my office complaining of a multitude of symptoms. Her neurological exam has a few subtle findings. I send her off to get a MRI scan of her head. It shows several bright spots, suggestive of the demyelinating plaques of multiple sclerosis. We do a spinal tap and the results come back positive for the markers of MS. I bring the patient back to review the test results. I worry about making her anxious before she can come in for her appointment. Hopefully she has someone to come with her with whom to share the information. Hopefully my schedule allows us to block enough time to answer all her questions without making her feel rushed. Hopefully we have had enough time during her earlier visits to have developed rapport. Hopefully she'll trust me. Hopefully she'll remember a third of what I have to tell her. Hopefully on her way in, she doesn't run into an acquaintance who has a niece whose boss's sister-in-law had the disease and ended up in a wheelchair within six months of diagnosis.

Seven years ago I would have told her that there wasn't too much to do except wait for another attack. It may come next week, next month, next year, next decade, maybe never. Today, we talk about immunomodulation, corticosteroids, the MS Society.

When Kim brought me *Women Living with Multiple Sclerosis*, I was thrilled to have another tool to offer my patients. Here was a chance to show my patients how other people, real people, lived with the disease. My copy of the book has become ragged, well thumbed through.

Living Beyond *Multiple Sclerosis* will inspire patients to transcend the effects of the disease and allow them to learn from others who have dealt with the disease with courage, attitude, and humor. It reflects the anger, denial, frustration, fear, camaraderie, courage, faith, resentment, and appreciation of life that my patients experience on a daily basis. This book will be a wonderful tool to offer my patients. To the wonderful, brave women who have poured their hearts and souls into these books, my eternal gratitude for helping me do my job!

Lily Jung, M.D., M.M.M.
PacMed Clinics

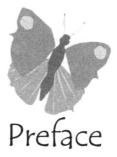

Preface

I t has been thirty years since the first signs and symptoms of multiple sclerosis showed up in my mind and my body. I went through years of absolute ignorance of what those signs and symptoms meant, more years of a "probable MS" diagnosis, to, seven years ago, finally seeing definitive proof on MRI films that the condition was, indeed, mine. It would seem that all that time, with all the physical, mental, emotional, and spiritual transmutations it effected, would have been enough for me to learn everything there is to know about living with the MonSter.

Even as I lived with It, though, I didn't comprehend the magnitude and complexity of what having MS meant. The medical texts that I read seldom described accurately any of my experiences. If I suspected that something that happened to me was somehow associated with MS, I couldn't find confirmation of that anywhere. I was sure that, besides having MS—or maybe rather than having MS—I was a freak.

Then, more than three years ago, I met a group of fellow female MSers on the MS message boards on America Online's AllHealth network. We got acquainted on the Mental Flutters Board (where we talked about the cognitive problems that come with MS) and moved from there to establish our own round-robin e-mail support system, the Flutterbuds Group, or the "Froup."

I was both dismayed and delighted to learn from these ladies that I wasn't alone. The strange happenings that took place every day in my being were not so strange after all, but were "gifts" from the MonSter that we all had in common. I was sorry that there were other people who had to deal with the same things, but elated to realize that I no longer had to deal with them alone.

Finally, there was a place where I could go to talk about the things that my doctors had never told me could be expected with MS and that nobody, myself included, would have believed had anything to do with MS. I could sympathize when one of the Flutterbuds talked about pain that made her want to rip her face off. I could laugh and cry when one of them wondered why her frozen pizza turned out soggy after she tried to bake it in the dishwasher. I knew that they identified with my claim that I could no longer sleep lying down and with my attempts to get my dog to obey commands by flicking the TV remote control in his direction. We, all of us, understood each other! We were finally free to discuss, honestly and intimately, the misadventures that come with living with multiple sclerosis. Best of all, we were free to react, honestly and intimately, to the MonSter's tricks.

We realized that what we'd found with each other was too good to keep to ourselves. We thought that other MSers might benefit from the knowledge that, no matter where they lived or what stage of the illness they'd reached, they had allies who battle the same adversary and who are willing to talk about it. We wanted to give readers with MS the assurance that the seemingly insignificant problems they encounter every day are, indeed, significant signs of the MonSter's work. We hoped to give readers without MS an inside look at what life with the MonSter entails. Those hopes and wishes led to the creation of *Women Living with Multiple Sclerosis*. In that first volume, the Flutterbuds talk mostly about the challenges we face as women with MS.

As we grew even more relaxed in our conversations, we began to concentrate less on trading lists of symptoms and the challenges they bring about and more on the ways we've devised to get past those challenges. We discovered, through our collective problemsolving, resources and strengths that we'd never suspected we had. We've survived the assaults of this Beast we call multiple sclerosis and have sometimes managed to outwit It along the way. We've come through each battle stronger, with our defensive skills sharpened. We've found serenity in the realization that sometimes it isn't even necessary to take up arms and fight. We only have to pick ourselves up and move beyond the battlefield. We've learned that, no matter what weapons the MonSter employs, It can't get to the inner parts of us. No matter how often or how severely It damages our bodies, It can't harm the elemental being in each of us.

One of the most valuable lessons we've learned since the Froup got together is that there are ways to get beyond barriers. Most of the time, the courage and ingenuity required to take us down the right path are within us. When we need directions, there are resources outside ourselves, willing to team up and travel with us. When all else fails, we can change the way we view the obstacles, redesign them if necessary, transform them from stumbling blocks into footholds. That's the message we hope to pass on to other MSers now.

As in *Women Living with Multiple Sclerosis*, most of what we discuss here is not based on medical or legal expertise. Even when we talk about giving ourselves injections or finding the right wheelchairs and canes or filling out forms for Social Security Disability benefits, we speak simply as women with multiple sclerosis who have done all these things.

We welcome the input, in several chapters, of Robert L. Reed, M.D., my neurologist (in my opinion, the best neurologist—for me, anyway. And, no, he didn't tell me to say that). He joins us, not to give medical advice, but to help us understand how we can best collaborate with medical caregivers to knock down the MonSter when that's possible or walk (wheel) around It when it's not.

Dedicated to the memory
of Russell, Loraine,
and Jim Swauger

Important Note

The material in this book is intended to provide anecdotal and personal information regarding multiple sclerosis. Professionals in the field may have differing opinions about this information and change is always taking place. Any of the treatments described herein should be undertaken only under the guidance of a licensed medical practitioner. The publisher, authors, editors, and professionals quoted in the book cannot be held responsible for any error, omission, outdated material, or adverse outcomes that derive from the use of any of these treatments or information resources in this book, either in a program of self-care or under the care of a licensed practitioner.

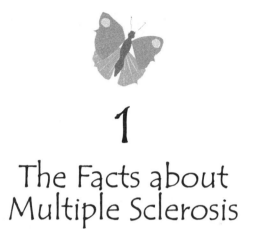

1

The Facts about Multiple Sclerosis

I'm somewhat uneasy about the title of this chapter. "Facts" makes it sound like what will be included is indisputable, with no questions attached. Some of the information here probably falls into that category; more of it comes from observation and speculation of researchers. As you read about what MS is, where it came from, and why it's here, keep in mind that this isn't a medical bible. Any statement which includes "may," "might," "sometimes," "usually," "typically," "perhaps," or any other indefinite description is subject to change as ongoing research separates facts from theories.

Multiple sclerosis (MS) is a disease of the central nervous system (brain and spinal cord). Onset of symptoms typically occurs between the ages of twenty and forty, although it has been diagnosed at earlier and later ages. Early signs and symptoms of MS may be so subtle they are ignored, attributed to exhaustion or general physical rundown, or dismissed as psychosomatic. Vision problems (blurred or double vision) are often the first sign that something is wrong. Other early symptoms may include numbness, tingling, and weakness in any part of the body. In some cases, loss of bladder and bowel control, lack of coordination, difficulty walking, slurred speech, difficulty swallowing, extreme fatigue, tremors, cognitive dysfunction, and emotional instability eventually show up. In severe cases, blindness and paralysis may occur. However, fewer than 25 percent of persons diagnosed with MS ever progress to a stage where they have to use a wheelchair all the time; even fewer are bedridden. Symptoms vary widely from one individual to another and, frequently, within one individual at different times. Even the most severe cases have been known to "burn out" unexpectedly, with the patient recovering to near-normal functioning.

Symptoms occur when the immune system attacks and destroys the myelin covering on nerve fibers within the central nervous system. The resulting inflammation and destruction of myelin—and, eventually, replacement of myelin with sclerotic (hardened) patches—interrupts messages to and from the brain.

More than 400,000 people in the United States have been diagnosed with MS. Worldwide, it is present in more than one million people. It is twice as prevalent in women as in men. The disease is not contagious. MS is not fatal; most people with MS have a near-normal life expectancy. Except for very rare cases, death associated with MS is from secondary symptoms, i.e., pneumonia, urinary tract infections, or skin breakdown in bedridden patients.

Although MS is not hereditary, a familial susceptibility has been observed. At least 10 percent of MSers have other family members with MS. People (especially women) who have a parent or sibling with MS have a 20 to 40 percent greater chance of developing the disease themselves. Thus, it's proven that there is some genetic link involved, but the strength of that link can't be measured as a single stimulus for acquiring MS. If genetics were the only factor, we could predict that, if one identical twin comes down with MS, the other would, too. Yet, in 70 percent of identical twins, where one has MS, the other doesn't.

This leads to the conclusion that several different factors must be present to produce multiple sclerosis.

Some authorities believe that a viral trigger is involved, based partly on the fact that outbreaks of MS have occurred subsequent to viral epidemics in areas where MS had been relatively unknown. It's also known that MS exacerbations frequently follow viral infections in individuals. Viruses that are responsible for measles, herpes, and any number of other conditions have been blamed for MS; further research hasn't turned up evidence that any of those are a direct cause.

There seems to be a relationship between geography and/or ancestry and the probability of having MS. It is most common among Caucasians of northern European heritage, while it's rare in Asians. People who spend the first fifteen years of their lives in tropical areas of the world are at significantly lower risk than the general world population; those who spend their first fifteen years in temperate regions have a greater risk. Changing locations after the age of fifteen doesn't make a difference; people retain their susceptibility relative to where they spent their earlier childhood years.

There is presently no cure for multiple sclerosis. However, since 1993, many new treatments have been developed which are proven to reduce the number of attacks and slow the progression of the disease. There are also many treatments available for symptomatic management of MS.

2

The Flutterbuds Are Back!

R eaders who have returned to listen in on more of the Flutterbuds' conversations will notice some changes in the Froup's roster. A few of our ladies have moved on to other pursuits since the publication of *Women Living with Multiple Sclerosis*. Several others are still official Froup members, but haven't been able to actively participate in our latest discussions. We've missed each of these friends and ask our guests to remember them, as we do, with fond thoughts.

At the same time, we welcome eight new voices to our circle of contributors. These ladies are members of another round-robin e-mail group, the Gutterbuds (the name was chosen only because it rhymes with Flutterbuds. Right, ladies?). Like the Flutterbuds, they met on the MS Mental Flutters Board in America Online's AllHealth area and broke away to form their own close-knit support network. For the sake of putting this volume together, we've merged to form a third group, The Flutterbuds Bookies. We're grateful for their generous and enthusiastic input.

Barb, one of the first Flutterbuds, is fifty-three. She was diagnosed with MS in 1995, then rediagnosed as suffering from spinal cord injury in 1998 at the Mayo Clinic. She is a good example of how difficult it can be to be diagnosed correctly. She and her husband, Charlie, have four children (youngest son, Tom, fourteen, still lives at home) and one grandson. The family moved from their farm in Texas to a ranch in Oklahoma in December 1998. Barb still works, but at a much less stressful job since their move. She plays the organ at her church every Sunday and believes that making time for her music has improved her physical condition.

Everybody needs a passion! Music is mine.

Bren is thirty-six years old and has remitting/relapsing MS. She lives with her significant other, Al; her daughter Sarah, twelve; and Al's son Kevin, ten. She has another daughter Kristina, fourteen, who lives with her father. An original Flutterbud, Bren's first MS attack after a six-year remission took place late in 1998; she had to use a cane for the first time then. Bren says that the last year has taught her to live with "new and annoying" symptoms. She recently began working part-time doing childcare at a health club, while doing a home-study course in medical transcription. She volunteers on America Online as an MS support chat host and as coeditor of a newsletter about MS.

I love helping folks with MS, even if it's just giving them a place to come and hang their hat for an hour or so. I can be reached at: hostahthbren@aol.com.

Bunny is thirty-five and is married to Paul. She has two "great" stepchildren, Jon-Paul, who is sixteen, and Taralyn, who is ten. Bunny is unable to work, but she blames that more on conditions (including a seizure disorder) other than MS.

I am in the "limbo" state of diagnosis. I've had symptoms of MS since 1992; I have three white spots on my brain, but it seems it's not enough for a diagnosis. So, I'm told it's all in my head. Yep! That's where the lesions are!

Chris, forty-eight (!), is married to Mike and has two grown sons, Andy and Adam, and a stepdaughter, Jill, who recently gave Chris and Mike their first grandson, Tyler. Chris was diagnosed with MS in 1995, after just three months of symptoms. The cognitive problems have been the hardest for her.

I started making mistakes at a job that I had held for twenty-two years, so I knew something was wrong! The hardest thing for me to do was to leave work and all my friends behind!!

Chris is one of the original Flutterbuds and is still known as "Ms. Excited," because she uses a lot of exclamation points in her letters (when we haven't stolen all of them from her!).

Debby is thirty-four and is married to Garth. They have four children; Jessica, fifteen; Amy, twelve; Ashley, nine; and little Jerry, seven.

My children are the reason I fight to not give in to the MonSter.

Debby also has three adult stepchildren: Jason, Shawn, and Melinda. Debby became a grandma at the ripe old age of twenty-seven and loves "every minute of it!"

Debby was diagnosed in 1998. What is her attitude toward MS?

With the love and support of my children and husband and with their ability to make me laugh and to not let me take myself too seriously, I am going to fight this thing every day. Each day is a new beginning, and my life has just begun.

Dee (who is really named Donna, a.k.a. Donna-Dee) is fifty-six. She is married to Al, and all of their children are grown (*and have blessed us with the most adorable grandchildren! But don't all grandparents say the same thing?*). It has been three years since Dee's "probable" MS diagnosis.

During that time, we have learned to live around the MS and with the MS. The MonSter does rear Its ugly head, and then we have to give

It our attention. But we survive and are stronger for it, maybe not physically, but certainly in other important ways.

Dev is forty-eight and has been married to Mike for twenty-eight years. She has three grown daughters, Stefanie, Vicki, and Patti; three grandchildren; and two step-grandchildren. Her last job was as an assistant to the owner of a group home for the elderly and mentally challenged. She stopped working in 1996. She was diagnosed with remitting/relapsing MS in 1988 after years of doctors telling her that her symptoms were psychosomatic. She has been in one of the Avonex® (one of the ABC drugs, the three most widely prescribed treatments for MS) studies since 1991 and credits her continued remitting/relapsing (as opposed to secondary progressive) status to that. She spends her time writing, drawing, trying new and unusual recipes, and fishing with Mike. Dev collects lighthouses and is "sort of a film buff."

One of my favorite sayings is, "If I can't make you laugh, then we'll cry together." The ladies in the group call me Dev except when I'm having a bad time and I'm feeling low. Then it's "Deedles."

Donna, forty-three, has been married to Gary for nineteen years. They have three children and six grandchildren, who all live nearby. She says that the time she and Gary spend with their family is the most satisfying part of their lives. She also has three stepdaughters and five step-grandchildren, whom she doesn't get to see as often as she'd like to. One of the first Froup members, Donna was diagnosed in 1997 and left her job as a police officer shortly after that. Several months after starting on one of the ABC drugs, her symptoms have eased enough to allow her to return to work in a civilian position on the police department.

I feel energized by the knowledge that I'm actively resisting the MonSter's assaults on my body and soul.

Helen is fifty-eight. She says that not much has changed since *Women Living with Multiple Sclerosis* was published.

I'm still with the same person [Janni, Helen's partner for the past seventeen years] *and still in the same house. The van and the dogs are different, but that's about all. The MS even seems to be about the same as always.*

Helen's worst problem is fatigue. We're not sure she can blame MS for that, since we've seen her stay up all night with sick puppies, construct insulated houses for stray cats, travel to visit her elderly aunt, and build computers; then she still finds the energy to tell us about it.

We've noticed that one thing about Helen has changed—she is no longer able to maintain her reputation as the Froup Curmudgeon. She tries, but we've gotten to know her too well to believe it.

Jamie (a.k.a. "Biker Babe") is (*almost!*) thirty-nine. She was one of the founding members of the Flutterbuds Group. She lives with her significant other, Jeff, and has a twelve-year-old daughter, Jaylon. She was diagnosed with MS in 1986, ten days after the onset of symptoms that were first identified as an ear infection, then as a stroke. After she recovered (better than expected!) from her first couple of attacks, she spent the next twelve years getting around with "*a walker on wheels, forearm crutches, a wheelchair, the walls and furniture, depending on what was available.*" [Jamie, you forgot to mention Harleys!] Jamie had several exacerbations last year which kept her hospitalized or in a rehabilitation facility much of the time. We've missed her in our online talks and are always happy and grateful to welcome her back when she's able to spend some time with us.

Janis (our "Rainbow" since the Froup began) is forty-four, married to Roger, with a daughter, Aleana, and a son, Joseph. She was diagnosed in 1996 and is now considered secondary progressive (one of the types or stages of MS, when remissions become fewer and less complete) but still uses just a cane to get around. One of her biggest problems is sensory overload.

I have what I call "freakin' & peakin'" times when too much is going on at one time.

We're not happy that Janis has this problem, but we love the way she describes it!

Joy, now fifty-nine, has had several visits from the MonSter since *Women Living with Multiple Sclerosis* was published. She says that she has been forced to curtail her activities accordingly, "*mostly in the realm of housework.*" Even so, she has managed to "be-bop" at high school reunions, care for four dogs, a cat, and several tanks of angelfish, and stay in touch with family and friends via e-mail. She is married to Jack and has a grown daughter, Jeni. Joy has been the Froup's "Saint" since we got together.

Karon hasn't grown up over the past couple of years; she's still our "Little Bit." She's married to Sal and has several stepchildren and a new granddaughter, Laney. For the past two years, she has traveled back and forth between Miami and Jacksonville, Florida, every other week to help her brother raise his daughter, Victoria. She says that the airport personnel now watch for her; they know what date it is by her flight pattern. Karon now uses a quad (four-legged) cane to help her walk.

At first it looked just functional; but I went to the craft store and got loads of stickers and dressed it up. I get lots of questions and compliments about it now. My new cane has given me lots of confidence. Slowly but surely, the black-and-blue marks from my many falls and spills (have you ever chased a two-year-old and not fallen?) are fading.

In *Women Living with Multiple Sclerosis,* Karon claimed to enjoy mostly solitary activities. With her new confidence, though, she says she's gotten out of her reclusive lifestyle and made new friends. She now belongs to two churches and one choir and attends many social functions.

Kat was known as Renee in *Women Living with Multiple Sclerosis.* She is married to Dewey and they have six grown children between them. They are now raising their grandson Derrick, who is twelve. Kat was the Flutterbuds' "Cybermom" who set up the round-robin forum we use in Froup communications. Kat has been uncharacteristically quiet during the past year; her mother and father both died recently. When she joins us now, it's usually to tell us a story about finding some new "little miracle"—a sign of God—working in her life.

Kathey is thirty-seven. She has one (*wonderful!*) son, Josh, who is seventeen.

She and her "fella," Kirk, have been in "one of those long-distance romances" for about three years. Kathey was diagnosed in January of 1999, the day after Josh's sixteenth birthday. Her first symptoms included a bout with optic neuritis (five years before her diagnosis) and facial numbness (two days before her diagnosis). She works nights as a registered nurse on a medical unit of a small hospital.

MS is not a death sentence, unless you let it be. Scary? You betcha. But the MonSter can give you a new perspective on what is truly important: Smelling the roses, petting a dog, hugging people, saying, "I love you," often and sincerely.

Kim (still our "Tinkerbelle"; we usually call her "Tink"), forty, was diagnosed ten years ago. She retired two years ago from her job as a nurse for Alzheimer's patients. She still lives with her dad and her brother Steve. She credits them and her friend Rita for getting her through each day. Kim spends most of her free time (*Let's face it—most of it is free time now!*) listening to her police scanner (her latest interest), developing websites, playing computer games, or visiting online with the Flutterbuds.

I have needed all the support I have received from them and have received all the support I needed. Without them, I would not be here now!

Laura, forty-two, is married to John. She began having recognizable MS symptoms on March 21, 1994, and was diagnosed on March 21, 1995.

March 21 is now known as "Laura Day." It's an annual holiday. If at all possible, I take the day off and do something fun or special for me.

It's been six years since I started with MS problems, and you would never know I have it. I really do "look so good." The thing I regret the most is my loss of innocence. You know that someday you will die or be ill or whatever, but that is far in your future, after a rich, full life. The MonSter can steal that idea from you, if you let It.

Laura is still able to work full time in contracting work for the government. She makes some of her own clothing, as well as elaborate costumes that she enters in competitions at costuming and science fiction conferences. She also helps run the conferences and collects vintage Barbie dolls.

Lori, one of the first Flutterbuds, is thirty. Lori was "possibly" undiagnosed with MS in 1998, after tests at the Mayo Clinic indicated that she probably has a still unnamed demyelinating condition similar to MS. Lori spends much of her time homeschooling her daughter Amanda. She is married to Steve.

Marge, our "Crone," is sixty-five. She and husband, Jerr, have several adult children. Diagnosed with MS in 1986, she also has fibromyalgia and several other autoimmune and allergic conditions. A heart attack in 1999 prevented her from being involved in most of our discussions since then. She spends a lot of time walking and carrying out the rest of her recovery regime.

Margo is forty-six. She was diagnosed with MS in 1998, after more than four years of going to different doctors and being told that there was "nothing wrong" and she should "consider counseling." She and her husband, Roy, have four daughters (two his, two hers), Cami, April, Michelle, and Holly and seven grandchildren. Margo retired from her job as a letter carrier in 1999, which, she says, made her redefine who she is.

I count my blessings now in different currency. I gauge my productivity by a different standard. It's been difficult to do this mental revamping, but even in my darkest hours, I have faith in my God, in my family, and in myself. I might not beat MS, but I will not let it beat me.

Nadiza is forty-seven. She is married to Joe, who, she says, can still make her laugh and feel young after twenty-six years together. They have two daughters, Nicole, twenty-two, and Allyson, twelve. Nadiza was diagnosed in 1988, when Allyson was only eight months old. We sometimes call Nadiza "Nature Girl" because of her love of plants, animals, insects, and the planet Earth in general. She has homeschooled Allyson since 1998, which she says gives her a chance to learn even more about nature.

Ramia was diagnosed in 1996 and is forty-one. She has been with the Flutterbuds since the group was formed. She and her husband, John, have two children, Brian, nine, and Haley, five.

Ramia's symptoms have gotten worse over the past two years, but she was still able to go on a ski trip and an Alaskan cruise. She started using a cane last year and recently got an electric scooter.

I do what I am able to do and try not to stress over things I can't control. I realize I am not God, so I just relax and go with the flow. If I were God, I'd get rid of this MonSter and all the other monsters in the world.

Robin, thirty-nine, is married to Patrick. They have three kids: Brandon, thirteen; Danielle, ten; and Jenna, three. She was diagnosed in 1998 and still works full-time as an executive assistant.

I try to take life a day at a time, and to say, "Thanks, God!" a lot. People tell me I'm nice. Ask my family whether I'm still "nice" after I've poured a few thousand milligrams of steroids into this body!

Sally, forty-eight, lives by the sea in California. She is an artist and has been doing most of her work with computer graphics. Her significant other is George, who lives in an apartment down the hall from hers. One of the original Flutterbuds, Sally is the owner of Sally's Fridge (from *Women Living with Multiple Sclerosis*), where all of the Froup members' lost remote controls, slippers, keys, and eyeglasses seem to end up.

My MS is fairly stable now and has been mostly quiet except for a few rough times with fatigue and sensory problems. I think I have put my MS in the Fridge for a while, instead of sending everything else I own there. I recently lost my purse and found it a month later in an ice chest/cooler. Does that count?

Sharon, forty-eight, is a social worker/psychotherapist and is presently the executive director of her county's Juvenile Court Diversion Program. Diagnosed as relapsing/remitting in 1995, she was recently reevaluated as secondary progressive. She married

Bob in 1998 in the living room of the house they'd just bought. This was the first Flutterbud wedding, with the Froup members serving as Sharon's cyber-bridesmaids.

Yes, Bob knew I had MS, but he married me anyway. He gets quite irate when people marvel over that fact. But I marvel over it, too!

Together Sharon and Bob are raising four teens, ranging in age from fourteen to nineteen. Sharon and Bob welcomed their first granddaughter, Madison Grace, daughter Leslie's baby, last year. Sharon is still our "Yankee Princess." At least we think that's what she's saying.

Tara, another original Flutterbud, is forty-four. She has three grown sons, Errol, Michael, and Jacob; one granddaughter; and a grandson on the way. Tara gave up her job as a special education consultant in 1998 because of progression of MS and a rare neurological disorder called Chiari malformation. She now works in Native American arts, designing and making prints, jewelry, and medicine bags. She also writes and illustrates children's books.

In 1999, the MonSter brought Tara a surprise benefit. A local newspaper ran a story about Tara's medical condition and her career change. She and Dean, the photographer who took her picture for the story, have been together since that day!

Vicki, forty-two, is still married to Larry. Their twins, Ash and Zach, are fifteen. Vicki also has a grown stepson, Jeremy. Thirteen years after her diagnosis in 1986, she was reevaluated as having secondary progressive/chronic progressive (a type of MS that has characteristics of two of the progressive types) MS.

But I still feel that every day that I wake up above ground is a good day.

I have to add myself in here. I'm Judy Lynn, Lynn, Judy, Judith, JL. It all depends on who is talking to me (or about me). I'm fifty-one and married to Ron (we just celebrated our thirtieth wedding anniversary!). Our daughters, Karen and Julie, are both grown and away from home now. Neither of them has seen fit to give me a grandchild yet. (I'm just stating a fact, girls, not nagging—I'm taking a two-minute break from that.) My physical condition, thirty years after the first symptoms of MS showed up, is not as good now as I'd hoped it would be, but much better than I'd expected it to be. Except for a few acute attacks, I've had only slow progression of the MS over the past ten years; that's been gradual enough to allow me to adjust as it happens.

I love my life. I have the *most wonderful* husband and family and lots of good friends. I'm never bored. I can't ask for more (unless it would be for a couple of grandkids—are the two minutes up yet?).

▲▲▲

Now that we've gotten to know each other, we'll talk for just a few minutes about what the Flutterbuds mean to each other.

Kathey Since I met the ladies in this Froup, I know that whenever I turn on my computer, there's a friend there ready to laugh or cry or just chat. I think of us as a combination of "Cheers" (where everybody knows your name, and they're always glad you came) and that song by the Eagles, about singing out loud the things we could not say. Together, we *sing*, girls!

Me I didn't realize what I was missing before I met all of you ladies. I didn't need a support group, or so I thought. Now I can't remember where I got that idea, or how I survived before I found out it was the *wrong* idea.

Helen Have you been reading my mind, Skinny Sister? I can't remember how I got by before, either. Now you gals are as much a part of my life as if you were blood kin, and I need you around!

Sally I feel the same way. I am a much happier person. I hardly ever have the deep bouts of depression I had before. The funny thing is that before I met this group, I didn't realize I was unhappy. I thought I was handling things well. Little did I know....

Joy Same here, Sally. Even before we officially started our group, when we were just talking on the Mental Flutters board, I found myself rushing to the computer every morning to read and post. I didn't think of my friends there as "a support group," just as a delightful bunch of women I enjoyed interacting with. The shared MS became one of many common bonds, rather than the *only* common bond. Our ability to joke about every aspect of our lives, including MS and the rest of the bad stuff, was really the strongest glue that bonded us. Do you remember how Kat drew us all into her web of craziness? She made it "okay" somehow to toss globs of purple gak against a wall or buy red wigs or pee on rocks or do whatever it took to keep laughing and to not take ourselves or life too seriously. I had never met anyone else quite like her, and I never will.

Dee Me, too! I remember noticing that she was gone from the Mental Flutters board, and so I wrote and asked her what had happened to her. She wrote me back and asked me to join the Froup, and the rest is history! Thank God for her!

Vicki I don't mean to downplay what y'all have meant to me for damn near three years now. But you are all so much more important now, if that's possible, since I am no longer working. Larry bought me this new computer, not because we needed it, but so I would have a more reliable way to keep in touch with y'all. Period. That's the only reason I have it. That was his idea, because he knows how much I need y'all.

Chris Here's my story about computers and Flutterbuds: My son Adam bought a computer, and it sat in our spare room for quite a while without anybody touching it! I swore I would never touch a computer at home. Who needed one? Well, when I wasn't able to work anymore, I finally decided to play around with it. I was then given a CD for AOL. I ended up on the MS message boards. Wow!!!!! What a find!!! People with MS, just like me!

When I was diagnosed, I knew nothing at all about MS! Talk about feeling scared! Then I met all my wonderful sisters. Living with MS has become easier just knowing that I am not alone with this MonSter anymore! I feel that there is nothing that MS can do to me now that I can't handle, because I have all of you here to help me.

Margo The things that we talk about are the kinds of stories I need to hear now and what I needed to hear in the beginning. I need to know that, just because my eyes are going kaputie on me now doesn't mean I'm doomed to blindness. I need(ed) to hear it from real, live people, not from doctors or agencies or other strangers. I can believe it if the information comes from people like me, just average MSers. I don't want to hear too much about the people that run marathons and stuff; they are the way-above-average exceptions to the norm. Aren't they? Or maybe I'm way below the norm.... I'm thrilled when I can manage to lift a gallon carton of milk to the shelf in the refrigerator.

Kathey If you are below the norm, so am I. But, hell! I couldn't run a marathon pre-MS! I know what you mean, though. I'd rather hear about folks living with MS the best they can, day to day. I'm proud of and thrilled for all the "wonder women" (and men) that I hear stories about, but I cannot identify with them. I prefer the kind of wonder women that we all are, struggling sometimes, but laughing and learning and sharing and loving and *living*.

Sharon Believe it or not, there are times when it's hard to belong to a group like this. Sometimes being involved in our conversations drains me. We discuss our loss and grief, our triumphs over this damned disease, its effect on our families, especially our kids. While you guys are writing, my mind is going a hundred miles-an-hour, reliving the diagnosis and the "old" days and remembering how it used to be before MS walked into my life. Writing to all of you and reading what you've written is a great way to get feelings out. But once they're out, they're so real and they create such emotion. The intimacy that comes with the sharing here is difficult. It makes it hard for me to pretend I'm okay.

Sally I have trouble with that too, Sharon. I feel like such a wimp when I whine. I feel I need to be strong for all of you folks, but I can't even be strong for me. When I feel bad, it's like I let all of you down, because I don't read fast enough to stay current. Then, when any of you needs something, I am too out of it to think of anything other than the same things I say all the time. But please know that when things are going rotten for you, I do say prayers and picture good things for you, even if I can't say it at the moment. I so admire all of you for being able to be there for each other. I feel like a taker, but I want to be a giver. How could you know the love I feel and the prayers I say for you when I am out of touch?

Helen Because we know *you*, Sally, m'dear, and we know all about that big wonderful heart of yours! You may think you don't give, but you do, just by being there and being yourself. You put so much caring into just a few words. Just accept the fact that we love you and are here for you, and then don't worry about it. We have all leaned on you at times, and you've been there for us, so now it's your turn to lean on us.

Dee Sally, when I read your note, all I could think of was that nothing of what you said about yourself is true! I think that all of us feel the way you do at one time or another. It is hard to always be able to come up with something significant to say. Sometimes I just read and pray, as you do. We all do that, depending on where our strength is at the time. You are a wonderful sister, and I always feel supported and loved by you!

Sally I do feel your support even when I can't offer any. Sometimes I wonder where I'd be if I hadn't met all of you ladies.

Helen I'm going to be selfish here and say that I wish we didn't have MS, but that we'd met each other anyway.

Me What else do we all have in common that might have brought us together? I can't think of anything. If we didn't have MS, would we have met at all? That's unthinkable! If it came to a choice between having both or not having either, I don't think I'd have a problem deciding. If having MS is part of the package of having you ladies in my life, then It's welcome.

Kat And this is exactly the reason I thank God everyday that I have MS. I've told a few people that I am grateful I have MS—they think I am totally deranged; I guess they attribute it to the disease. My personal opinion is that all of us, this whole group, together and individually, have more smarts than most, because we learn from each other how to get along every day with the MonSter, who is very hard to get along with! I believe we look deeper, seek more knowledge about everything and everyone in our lives because we know, from knowing each other, that there is good everywhere. We are in a position to teach people compassion, because we've learned it right here with each other.

What I'm trying to say is that having MS is yet another sign that God is working in my life. Sure, he could have brought us together under some totally different circumstances. Who knows? Who cares? Not me. I just know that, as ugly as the MonSter is, It screwed up and sent me many blessings—y'all! And I bet that pisses It off big time!

Dee Although I would never choose to have MS or want anyone else to have it, I am blessed because of MS. Having this superb group of sisters as support is a transforming grace in my life and soul. I am also deeply thankful for the faith we all share. We rarely have the same beliefs and ideas about religion, but we share the same inner commitment to one another. We pass this strength on to one another and back again. We know it is not for us alone. One of the reasons for writing this book is that we want to share this strength with others.

Sharon Friends are angels who lift us to our feet when our wings can't remember how to fly. Everything considered, this is how I feel about all of you!

Amen, Sharon!

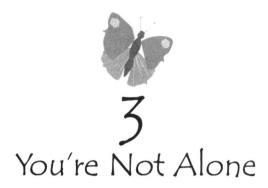

3
You're Not Alone

This chapter is a message to readers, especially those newly diagnosed who might be having a hard time with the whole concept of having multiple sclerosis. Let's say you are a member of the "newbies" group. Your doctor has just told you that you have MS. You're being inundated with information and advice, solicited and otherwise. You're trying to sift through the mishmash of facts about MS that you know for sure, of tales about the doom and destruction of body and mind and spirit that you expect to soon experience for yourself, and of disbelief that this could be happening to you. You're angry, depressed, and confused. You might even be relieved (and astonished at your relief!) that what you have is MS, rather than any number of other conditions that were on your "maybe I have..." list. You might feel validated in the knowledge that what you have is a real, physical, medical disorder. From now on, nobody can tell you that you've imagined all your symptoms, that you've brought them on yourself, and that if you'd just concentrate on something else/make up your mind to get better/remember how lucky you are/pray about it, you'll be fine. But the one feeling that underlies, wraps around, and ties together all the other emotions is fear. You want to know more about MS, but that will mean confronting the power of the MonSter, looking It straight in the face while It taunts you with what It can do to you. You want to talk with others who have the condition, but you're afraid that if you associate with them, admit that they're your peers, you'll end up with all the same disabilities that they have.

Maybe you're not a "newbie." Maybe you were diagnosed with MS many years ago. It's probably hard to admit that you're still (or again) going through the same emotional jumble that you "should" have sorted out at the very beginning. MS can make you feel that you're starting from scratch with the idea of getting used to it every time a new symptom shows up or worsens or disappears or reappears. Once again you're terrified of what you know can happen or what you think will happen.

The good news is that, if you've opened this book of your own free will, you've already taken a big step toward getting over the fear. You're saying that you want to know what you have to know. As you read these discussions that have taken place among nearly thirty women with MS, you'll learn firsthand about the rotten things that the MonSter can do to you. You'll also be assured that It can't overcome Its captives completely or for long. The ladies in the Froup have collectively lived through just about every kind of assault that the Beast can conjure and we're still around to talk about it. Sometimes we even laugh about it. In the talking and the laughing and the sharing of ideas and tips, we've found ways to survive Its antics and, sometimes, even to thrive on them.

Some of the Flutterbuds have had MS for several decades. Others aren't even sure that they have MS. No matter how long you've lived with the MonSter, there's somebody here who knows what you're going through. Our goal is to offer help and hope to other MSers, to let them know that they're not alone, and to share some of the weapons that we've found most effective in this great war (and in the little daily battles) with the Beast.

To begin with, some of the Flutterbuds look back on what it was like to hear that diagnostic dictum, "You have multiple sclerosis." Remembering that mixed-up time, they give a few words of advice to other MSers, newly diagnosed or veterans, who have decided to travel with us through this book.

▲▲▲

Kim The first bit of advice I can offer is, don't listen to what everybody is going to tell you about MS from now on. You'll hear that awful things are going to happen to you. That is not always the way it is. When I was diagnosed, I had a great doctor who stressed that the worst is not what always happens, or even what happens most of the time.

Even so, the frame of mind I was in when I got the diagnosis did not allow me to truly hear what the doctor was saying. So take a friend, spouse, brother, or sister to go with you when you see your doctor. The first few times you go, you will be overwhelmed. It's nice to have a second pair of ears to catch what you miss. Then keep on living. Don't throw in the towel. The cure might show up tomorrow! Hang around and see!

Laura Don't be scared by the crap you see about how debilitating MS is. I can't deny that I wonder about what tomorrow holds for me. But five years after my diagnosis, six years after I noticed the first symptoms, and ??? years after the MonSter sneaked into my life, I still "look so good." I just spent a week walking (yes, walking! even if I did use the cane occasionally) around Disney World. My brain is still sharp, too, sharper than a lot of completely "healthy" brains.

MS is not a death sentence. It's a life alert. It's a chance to be made aware of the choices you may need to make for the rest of your life and to be prepared.

Nadiza My advice to the newly diagnosed would be to educate yourselves about the disease from a variety of sources. People with MS have to look beyond what our doctors tell us and to remember that many doctors are as ill-informed about MS as most people in the general population are. Don't shut yourself off from the world. Somebody out there has gone through this before you; the load is easier to carry if you allow somebody to share it with you. Above all, keep your sense of humor. Dealing with the attacks of the MonSter is much easier if you can find a reason to laugh about it.

Dev   Be honest with your loved ones. They aren't going to know how you feel unless you tell them. One of the biggest mistakes I made was to not tell my family and friends how I felt about having MS. I've found that being honest about what I'm going through has eliminated a lot of the guilt feelings that I used to have when I wasn't able to accept every invitation I'd get. I used to think it would be an imposition on my friends and family to have small functions at my place (instead of huge gatherings elsewhere), and include everyone in the planning, preparation, and, of course, the cleanup. But they're happy to do whatever they can to help. I think it makes them feel that they are doing something to help me beat the MonSter! Do what you can, when you can do it. If you don't get it done, don't beat yourself up over it; just do it another time when you feel up to it.

Don't apologize for having a bad day. Even people who don't have MS have bad days.

Vicki   Allow yourself to mourn your losses, but remember that, most of the time, the losses are temporary. Above all, remember that if a symptom does not remit, you are no less a person because of it. I saw a movie tonight with a line in it that I think fits. "Dumbo still flew without his feather." So can we.

Bren   Remember that not everybody with MS experiences the same symptoms, and it almost never happens that somebody with MS gets all the possible symptoms. Learn all you can about the disease, but don't let it scare you.

Find a neurologist whom you trust and can talk to, and,

most importantly, one that listens. Don't let him/her brush you off, simply because he/she may not have heard of a particular symptom being caused by MS. If your neurologist is unavailable to speak with you on the phone or does not return your phone calls (or at least have the nurse return them), then you need to find another one.

Jamie Do not 1) believe everything that one doctor says—get a second opinion; 2) believe everything that you read or hear about MS—no two cases are alike; 3) let other people's reactions be a source of your stress—the less stress that you subject yourself to, the better the MS will be; 4) let anybody tell you that what's wrong with you is all in your head—you're the only one who knows how you feel!

Bunny Even though we share many of the same symptoms, we're still capable of doing different things. There are going to be good days and bad days, so expect to take each day as it comes. When I found out it was possible that I have MS, I did a lot of research. I didn't want the doctors knowing more than I do about me. I didn't want to live my life on the basis of what might happen to me. I'm glad I educated myself, because now I know that I most likely will not be that "drooling person" in the wheelchair.

Robin Stay in tune with your body. Pay attention to what it tells you. It will take time to learn to differentiate between "normal" body stuff and MS involvement. This was the biggest adjustment I needed to make and the one I still struggle with—matching what my body tells me with what my mind wants to do, then coordinating it all so I can do more, rather than less. Think efficiency!

The MonSter is just a resident in your body. How you choose to live with it is still up to you. The inner part of you, your spirit and soul, does not get touched by the MonSter. This most vital part of you is what can give you the strength you didn't know you had to keep on living a full, happy life. Be open to new possibilities, keep a positive outlook, and pray that the researchers will find a cure tomorrow!

Helen Never give up. Having MS isn't any fun, that's for sure. But it's not terminal and not always horrible. It seems to come with its own built-in strength to help you through the bad days. Go about your life as though every day is going to be a good day. When the days are good, rejoice. When they aren't, say your equivalent of "Oh, shit!" and wait for the good days to come back. Ninety percent of the time, they will. Don't feel weak or guilty when you have a "pity party" day. We all need and deserve one occasionally. Just don't let it become a way of life. Be willing to pick yourself up, dust yourself off, dry your eyes, and go on from there.

Keep a positive attitude. That way, the good days will be better, and the bad days won't be so bad. Think of the attitude you see in the dachshund that attacks the German Shepherd—it may get knocked on its ass, but it gave it a good shot!

Kat Savor each moment for the precious gifts that we have been given, and don't pass up a chance to do something, anything, that will help someone else with MS. As we've found out, in helping others, we help ourselves.

Tara Hiding what you are dealing with only makes others feel confused or shut out. That doesn't mean you have to go around handing out pamphlets. Just talk about the things that happen to you. Once others know that it's okay to discuss MS and see that you treat it in a matter-of-fact way, they'll relax and go along with your attitude. If somebody close to you will not be educated, refuses to discuss MS with you, or is critical of how you handle life, remember it's that person's issue, not yours!

Ramia No matter how hard it is to accept a diagnosis of MS,

don't be afraid to start on one of the ABC drugs as soon as possible. Make sure you find a doctor you have faith in, feel comfortable with, and like. Read, read, read, and share what you learn with your doctor. He or she may not know as much as you do about some things.

Debby We all must go through the grieving process; don't be surprised if you've already gone through one stage, like anger, and it comes back again later. Every day will bring a new and different awareness and a new acceptance of who you no longer are, of who you are now, of who you are still becoming. You might have to go through one or another stage of acceptance every day.

Chris As you read the rest of this book, you might see something about MS that scares you. That does not mean that it will happen to you!!!! Just read the book, keep the information you need, chuckle at the things that you find funny, and toss everything else over your shoulder!!!!

Kathey Read all you can about MS. Scour the Internet, the public library, the local hospital's library, bookstores, anywhere. But make sure the information you find is up-to-date. Keep in mind that our understanding of MS is much different now from what it was even five years ago. Treatment options are much better now. Remember that just because a doctor calls himself "Doctor MS" doesn't mean that he always knows what's best for you. Just because somebody says, "I was cured by eating only cardboard for seventeen months and three days," doesn't mean it will work for you or that it won't hurt you.

Ask lots of questions. Don't hesitate to stop a doctor or a nurse and say, "Wait, please explain that again or write it down for me."

As you learn all this information, pass it on! Tell your friends, family, coworkers, neighbors about MS. Knowledge is power. Misconceptions about MS come from folks just like us who don't want to say "I have multiple sclerosis" and explain what that means.

Laugh. Then laugh some more. Laugh so hard you pee your pants, then laugh because you peed your pants. Cry. Then cry some more. Cry so hard you pee your pants, then cry because you peed your pants. Then laugh because you've got snot all over your face from crying.

I guess the point is, take it all in and then let it all out! There are no guarantees, negative or positive, with this Beast. You can still make your life whatever you want it to be.

Vicki My first neurologist told me about his first MS patient, who died when he was sixty-seven years old. He had a heart attack on the tennis court! Don't let stupid or insecure people tell you how to manage MS. Don't let "what ifs" control what you do or don't do!

Joy MS is like a bear: unpredictable. Just as most wilderness hikers and campers escape injury from grizzlies, so do most people with MS escape the worst attacks of the MonSter. On your journey into these unfamiliar forests, arm yourself with knowledge of the Beast. Take savvy companions along with you: physicians, friends, family members, therapists. They will help you find the right path, provide you with the defense weapons you need, and surround you with warm light when the night is cold and lonely.

Allow yourself to be encouraged by the uncertainty of an MS diagnosis. The dangers are real, but so are the reasons for hope.

Believe in your own courage, and enter the woods smiling.

As you go through this book and read about how other people face the hurdles that MS throws in our paths and, more often than not, find ways to get past them, you're going to say, "But that's not me. That person doesn't have the same problems, the same circumstances, the same strengths or weaknesses, hopes and dreams, disappointments and frustrations that I have. I can't handle it that way." That's true! My advice is to follow your own timetable. You know what you're able to do, and you'll know when the time is right to do it. Learn from others who have gone down the same path, but don't necessarily try to keep pace with them.

Someday, maybe a month from now, maybe thirty years from now, you'll be able to look back at the days you've spent with MS. You'll recall times that you found new solutions to old problems, got up when you thought you'd fallen for the last time, took one more step when you thought you'd run out of road. You'll realize that, no matter how closely the MonSter trails you, It isn't powerful enough to capture you. You'll understand when somebody says, "I have MS; It doesn't have me." And you won't be able to keep yourself from sharing that message with others who have just been told that they have MS.

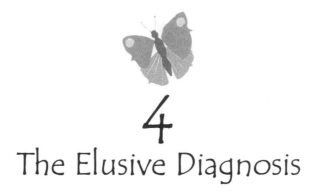

4

The Elusive Diagnosis

It's Sally's birthday. We start out as any group of friends would, wishing her the best. As usual, we don't stay on one track in our conversation for very long.

Bren   Happy birthday, darlin'! Don't forget to check your fridge. Maybe somebody "lost" a cake, and it'll turn up there.

Me   I don't think so, Bren. Old slippers? Car keys? Coffee cups? That's the kind of stuff that ends up in Sally's fridge. But birthday cakes? We eat those so fast, they don't have a chance to get lost. But, Sally, if you find my yellow robe in the fridge, send it back, and I'll bake you a cake, okay? In the meantime, have a happy birthday!

Dee   Yes, have a great day, Sally. Happy birthday, you old coot!

Sally   Watch it, Dee. People who call me names don't get any cake. I have other ways of getting even, too. Do you want me to get out my magic doll and put the pins back in the places that make you choke?

Bren   Oh, Dee, be careful! Sally, you can do things like that? Well now, that explains why my hemorrhoids are acting up lately. You're the culprit!

Me Has anybody ever considered the possibility that none of us has MS? We each just did something in a previous life to piss Sally off, and she's still trying to get even.

Sally That must mean that I pissed myself off too. Come to think of it, I do that on a regular basis anyway. But why would I want to get even with myself?

Joy Interesting notion, Lady Lynn. I guess we're lucky, though. Now, if it was Helen we had pissed off in a previous life, we'd all be dead by now.

Me I doubt it, Joy. Helen wouldn't let us off that easy.

Helen You got that right, Honeychile! I only wish I could remember what I did to Sally to make her so mad at me. Maybe it had something to do with the cattle I "borrowed" from that ranch back in 1850? Were those yours, Sal? How long are you going to hold a grudge?

Barb I can't remember what I did either, but I guess I didn't make her as mad as some of you did. She took the spell off me! No more MS—just dumb symptoms. Actually, I am ever so thankful at how well I'm doing. It's been a whole year already since I went to the Mayo Clinic and got my "undiagnosis." That's hard to believe. Time passes so quickly at my age.

And at Sally's age, even faster! Oops! Was that a pinprick I felt?

Donna Time does go by fast. Dee and I were both diagnosed in 1997. It seems like yesterday.

Vicki I bet they even used those new-fangled, fancy MRI machines to diagnose you two. Way back when I was diagnosed, I had to go through the carry-on baggage x-ray machine at the airport. The times, they are a-changin'!

Donna   Now I'm jealous. You got to ride the conveyor belt!

Vicki   There was a conveyor? I had to crawl very slowly through it. The conveyor must have a weight limit.

Kim   You're still lucky, Vickers. I was diagnosed so long ago, they just made me shake my head hard and listened for a rattle.

▲▲▲

Yes, we're joking. We realize that any Psychology 101 student would have a field day with our exchanges. We're laughing about something that's deadly serious, a diagnosis of multiple sclerosis. Sometimes it's easier to joke about our slides into denial than to admit, even to each other, even to ourselves, that the truth can be overwhelming. At other times, humor doesn't fit the mood. And the "mood" might hit long after disbelief should have stopped being an issue.

▲▲▲

Me   Do we ever get used to the idea that, whether or not we did something to make Sally mad, we really do have MS? I went through almost five years of hoping that somebody could tell me what was wrong with me. Then I had sixteen years of "probable MS" status, of the "maybe" and "maybe not" sides of my brain trying to outdo each other. Finally, I had an MRI. I looked at the white spots all over my brain on the film, and said to Dr. Reed, "So, there really is MS there?" He said, "Lots of MS, unfortunately." There I had it. "Definitely" had won over both kinds of "maybe." I'd seen the evidence with my own eyes, heard the interpretation and diagnosis with my own ears, from a doctor I trust completely. Yet, once in a while, there's still something inside me that says, "Maybe he read it wrong. Maybe the film was defective. Maybe I'm just a total screwup and everybody's still trying to placate me with a snow job."

Kim   You know, I am the same way, JL. I didn't see my MRI, but I do have a hard copy of the report. Sometimes I have to pull it out and make sure the information is right, that it's really my name and my doctor's name and my date of birth on it. I am sure that I am starting to grow into the MRI results, which doubly pisses me off! This isn't an easy thing to accept! You'd think we'd be pros at it by now!

Maybe we still go through times of uncertainty so that we can listen with a bit of sympathy and understanding to our MS buds who are still "actively" seeking an explanation for their problems.

Bunny   You know, when we're faced with the possibility of having this MonSter, why do we have to wait so long to find out definitely? I have the symptoms; I have three white spots on my MRI; I still don't have a diagnosis. It's so frustrating!

Me   I don't understand why three white spots would not be diagnostic of MS. What's your doctor waiting for, Bunny?

Bunny   The MRI results stated that there are three tiny areas of increased signal in the white matter. They say these findings are nonspecific and can be seen with areas of demyelination, changes from migraine, or other causes. So, basically, he's waiting for more conclusive "clinical findings," such as a positive spinal tap. My last spinal tap was normal, with the exception that the "demyelination count" was lost. I'm so frustrated!

Joy   It's like when I joked after my first MRI, which showed only one spot, that I had "singular sclerosis" instead of multiple. I was fortunate (?) enough to have a long history of MS-like symptoms, plus current symptoms that were typical of MS, with other possible causes ruled out. I can understand your frustration, Bunny, but from what I've read, your doctor is not alone in the way he approaches a diagnosis. It seems that, for many people, it's a "wait and see" kind of thing that can keep you in limbo.

Kim   I bet you are frustrated, Bunny. I'm sure someone already asked this, but is there any chance that you could see another neurologist?

Bunny   Yep, it's been asked, and it's been done. I've been to two university hospitals. The doctor at one said I was completely psychotic. The doctor at the other says there is definitely something neurologically wrong and that my neurologist should follow up with six-month checkups.

Kim   Is there any way that you could go back and see this second guy again?

Bunny   He doesn't want to see me again till I'm confirmed as having MS. He is a specialist for MS only, and he doesn't treat patients until they're definitely diagnosed.

Robin   So keep going back to your regular neurologist! Make a pest out of yourself. Report everything new that happens. You told us that he ordered steroids for you, in case your symptoms are caused by inflammation. Keep him informed on the progress with those, too!

Bunny   Oh, Robin, don't worry, I will report back to him. In fact, even though he doesn't want to see me for six months, he said just what you said; that once I finish this round of steroids I should call him and let him know my progress. I'm most definitely going to be a pest!

Bunny was true to her word. I doubt that she made a pest of herself, but she tried.

Bunny I did go back to my oh-so-humble (not!) neurologist and was pleasantly surprised! The scoop is, although my neurological exam this time was actually better on some points, my balance is worse, and he didn't like a couple of other things that he saw. He said there's definitely something wrong neurologically!

Me Bunny, this is so funny/sad to hear you say that you're pleasantly surprised that the doctor really thinks something is wrong. So he thinks that something is going on besides what's actually visible on your MRI? I wonder, does this mean that sometimes the MRI isn't the be-all/end-all for figuring out what's wrong?

Tara Some doctors would agree with that. My neurosurgeon says that he thinks that there is too much weight put on MRIs. He says he gets frustrated when doctors tell patients they definitely don't have MS, based on lack of lesions on an MRI.

Karon Some people have such mild MS that they don't have visible lesions. They just have bunches of symptoms. That's how I got my diagnosis; my MRI never did show any lesions. It takes a brave neurologist to diagnose definite MS without any test results to back it up.

Kim Sometimes lesions are present that are not visible on MRI. They are picked up much later, on autopsy.

Karon That's what I heard too, Tink. The big joke in my family is that they'll never know what's really wrong with me until the autopsy results are in.

Before MRIs were in common use as diagnostic tools for MS, many of us heard that line about ourselves. Thankfully, none of us was in that much of a hurry to get a definite diagnosis. Often, though, a diagnosis is delayed by our own belief, or that of the doctors we consult or the people who see us every day, that our symptoms originate in our minds, rather than in our brains and spinal cords. Once we get into that frame of mind, it seems futile to keep looking for other names to give to our array of symptoms. It's no wonder that Sally gets the voodoo dolls out when we talk about diagnosing MS. Here's her story:

Sally I was diagnosed in 1982, but have had symptoms since 1969. At that time I lost the vision in the left half of both eyes for a little over a day. The Cleveland Clinic did many tests, including a pneumo-encephalogram, which left me with an air bubble in my head for a few months. Over the next few years I had various transient troubles: overwhelming fatigue, weakness, tingling and pinpricks [not the voodoo kind] in my right leg, more eye trouble, a feeling that I had poured boiling water on several different areas, numb spots here and there. None of this really interfered with my daily life or lasted long enough for me to seek medical attention. I thought it was "all in my head."

In 1975, I was assaulted and spent six weeks in the hospital with very weak legs, eye trouble, and a concussion. I was tested and retested for spinal cord damage, until I couldn't stand it anymore and asked to go home. Over the next few months I got back to walking without crutches through sheer willpower. I started having more sensory problems with my leg and was referred to a neurologist. Because he didn't acknowledge that there even was a problem, I was more certain than ever that it was all in my head. In 1981 I lost the central vision in my right eye. The eye doctor referred me to a new neurologist, who did more tests and gave me the tentative diagnosis of possible MS. Several more episodes of eye trouble, hospitalizations, adrenocorticotropic hormone (ACTH) treatments and tests led to the diagnosis. In many respects it was a relief to know that there was a physical cause and that I wasn't just "cracking up."

Bunny While we're talking about this, I need to mention something else that bothers me. I was at a friend's house yesterday (who, I might add, is the one who first suspected I might have MS). Anyway, I brought information about Montel [Williams, who revealed his MS diagnosis in 1999] for her to read, which she found very interesting. But her husband made a comment that really hurt me. He basically said that I "look for things wrong" with me, that I should "just stop going to the doctors and forget about all this." He is convinced that I sit here and make up all these symptoms, then self-diagnose them. I love this couple dearly. But I keep hearing his words over and over in my head.

Me Bunny, does this guy care as much about you as you do about him? It sounds like he's letting fear speak for him. He knows you're not making anything up, but he doesn't want to admit it. If he did, that would mean that he agrees that there is something wrong.

Bunny I think he does care for me, JL. He and his wife have stuck by us through lots of trouble. Maybe you're right and it is fear talking. But he made me feel like that one neurologist did, that I'm psychotic and should be institutionalized!

Kathey Psssst, Bunny! Maybe he's related to that neurologist? Tell him that if you were going to invent symptoms, you'd choose nymphomania instead. It's more fun.

Bunny Anything would be more fun than this. My neurologist said if I do have MS, I'm in the early stages. If this is the early stages, ouch!

Nadiza I don't believe in "stages." I think that with MS, it's more like it's either mild or severe. I have had MS for at least twenty years and was diagnosed nearly eleven years ago. I am still doing better than you are, Bunny. I have never needed a wheelchair. I have used a walking stick for hikes, but I have never needed a cane. I did not consider myself to be in the early stages eleven years ago; I do not consider myself to be in the early stages now. I did and do believe that I have a relatively mild form of MS, with no stages involved.

Bunny   What was it like for you when you were going through all of this?

Nadiza   I waited four and a half years for a diagnosis. I saw a number of different doctors, and I ran the gamut of hearing how it was all in my head, how I was worrying too much, how I had lots of issues in my past that needed to be addressed. The neurologist's wife was the psychologist who tested me. I think since they couldn't figure out the organic cause, they decided they'd rake in the dough with psychological fees. MS was never mentioned as a possibility until three days before I was actually diagnosed. Before that, I thought I was going to die any minute from whatever it was that was wrong with me. MS as a possibility would have been a welcome alternative to the world of the total unknown that I was in. The time between Allyson's birth and the diagnosis eight months later was the worst. I cried for Nicole losing her mother so young and I cried for Allyson because I thought she would never have a memory of me. I hated the unknown more than anything else.

The final insult was that the doctor I was seeing diagnosed me as having a bladder infection. Joe recognized that I didn't have any of the symptoms of a bladder infection. It was at his insistence that I went to another doctor. Eight days after seeing Dr. Itsa Bladderinfection, I saw Dr. I. Listento Mypatients, a.k.a. Dr. Kovacich. He referred me to Dr. Caresabout M.S. Patients, a.k.a. Mridula Prasad, M.D. Dr. Prasad is the one that finally ended my search into the unknown and put my mind at rest about whether I needed to be in the looney bin.

Dev Oh, I know exactly how you felt, Nadiza, and you too, Bunny and Sally. I was having problems for years and went to so many doctors. They told me it was all in my head. After about four years of constant tests, I was ready to give up. Then I had a horrible attack and landed in the hospital. They even called Mike to the hospital at 3:00 one morning, because they thought I was having strokes and wasn't going to make it. That was as far as they went with a diagnosis. I was sure I hadn't had any strokes. I always suspected MS because we have so many people in my family with it. But, all the doctors said, "Oh, no, that's not it." I can't begin to list all the things they told me it might be.

I think I was barely sane. I just felt helpless, and I thought no one wanted to help me. Most of my thinking was along the lines of "where do I go from here?" As you know, everything that is suspected goes into your file, and every doctor I went to wanted the file from the previous doctor. They all pretty much said the same thing, that it was psychosomatic. I refused to give up. I called Cleveland Clinic and got a wonderful neurologist who actually listened to me. Within a week I had a diagnosis of MS. It just burns me up to think that there are others that are having problems like I was having and are being told it's psychosomatic. I've talked to people that went even longer without a diagnosis. It's a shame.

Dr. Reed offers us some explanations for delays in the diagnosis of MS and why the patient and the doctor (surprise!) can both become frustrated along the way.

Dr. Reed Fifteen to 20 percent of patients with any chronic disease have symptoms years before a definitive diagnosis can be made. The symptoms are often vague without specificity, and initial testing is often negative. This is the breeding ground for unhappy patients and perplexed doctors.

Let's review two patients who go to their doctors with very real symptoms. The first patient presents with blindness and pain in one eye. In this case, the doctor can perform a simple test, and optic neuritis [a common first symptom of MS] is confirmed immediately. A diagnosis of MS is likely, a plan for the future can be structured, treatment initiated.

The second patient says, "Doctor, I'm so tired, I can't go to work, and my feet tingle all the time." The exam results may be normal, as well as high-tech studies such as MRI and spinal tap. This patient may need to wait for a new set of specific symptoms with objective findings at the time of the examination before the doctor makes a definitive diagnosis.

Many symptoms, doctor visits, and tests later, patient and doctor become frustrated. The doctor may become less sensitive to the patient's concerns as time goes by ("I just did those tests last month, and here you are again with the same complaint!"). This leads to patient frustration and loss of confidence. So the patient sees a new doctor or several new doctors. The doctor the patient is seeing at the time a test finally confirms the diagnosis is the savior. ("Why couldn't that incompetent, insensitive first doctor have made the diagnosis two years ago and saved me all this time, pain, expense, and worry?")

Sometimes the doctor infers that, since the tests are not diagnostic, the symptoms are unreal. That is usually far from the truth. It helps if he or she explains that it takes time for the symptoms to develop to the point of a definitive diagnosis. Timing of tests is crucial. It is important to avoid early testing when symptoms are vague and the examination is normal. Negative tests reinforce the concern that these symptoms are really "in my head." Early testing is often painfully unrevealing and disappointing to the patient. The doctor should help the patient to understand the need to test at the opportune time. If the patient and doctor can communicate their frustrations during the process, it can work to the satisfaction of both.

Debby My neurologist hasn't officially documented that I have MS. He's waiting until I have insurance. He said if he made a diagnosis before I got insurance, I could forget getting coverage. So, for now, he's just documenting symptoms, like weak legs, weak eyes, etc. Not many doctors would do that for a patient.

Kathey I have a diagnosis, but my doctor is waiting to document the type of MS I have. It seems I'm picking up symptoms like a danged freight train since last year. We talked about doing another MRI, to check for possible brainstem-area lesions. But then the neurologist said, "Wait! We can't take a chance on the insurance company labeling you as a progressive 'type' until they're willing to pay for treatments for that as well as they do for remitting/relapsing."

Kathey's doctor's comment brings up another good point about diagnosis of multiple sclerosis. Even after the presence of MS is confirmed, there is almost always another (sometimes long) period of time before the type of MS (remitting/relapsing or one of the progressive types) that is present can be determined. That can make a big difference in the way the doctor treats the MS, in the way the insurance company covers the costs of treatments, and in the way the patient views herself and plans for her future. So a diagnosis doesn't necessarily mean the end to questions about what's going on.

Bunny I've only been at this search for a couple of years. But is there anybody else here who is still struggling as I am for a diagnosis? I mean besides just holding back for insurance purposes? Am I alone?

Jamie Don't fret, Bunny—before we met you, some of us Flutterbuds were diagnosed, then undiagnosed, then told that "MS can't be ruled out completely." We know you have something like MS, because you fit in so well with us!

Dee Bunny, I don't have a firm diagnosis, either. Mine is a "probable MS" verdict. I just don't worry about it anymore. I believe what I have is MS and fibromyalgia. I don't see how it could be anything else. The doctors believe this, too. Like you, I lack a "definite MS" MRI report. Mine says "cannot rule out demyelinating disease."

I hope this helps, at least a little bit, to make you feel less alone.

Barb I knew for two years that I had MS, because the doctor said so. Now I know I don't have MS, because another doctor said so. Who do I believe?

I was first diagnosed in 1995, after years of symptoms, tests, tears, and hair pulling. The neurologist in Texas, where I lived at the time, had run the usual battery of tests: MRI, CT scans, evoked potential tests (where they stick the needles on your legs to check for neural response times), and, of course, the ongoing walk-with-one-foot-in-front-of-the-other-and-watch-me-fall-over tests.

As the symptoms increased, so did the medications, of course. There were pain medications, medicines to help with bladder control, to relieve anxiety and spasms, and to help with balance problems.

In 1998 I went to the Mayo Clinic. They repeated all the tests I'd had over the past four years, along with some cognitive function tests (which I was sure I'd failed, but which I passed with flying colors!). Anyway, the doctors determined that most of my symptoms were from degenerative arthritis of the spine, scar tissue on my spine from an old injury, and all the medicines I was taking. The bladder problem was mostly from being forty-something and having had several kids. The cognitive problems are just that—little flutters that everyone has. I think I have that worse than most people, but I have learned to cope by being very regimented. That's not hard to do, since I tend to be anal retentive anyway!

I had to be weaned off the medicines, and about eight weeks after that my balance was so much improved and the spasms eased so that I didn't need to use my cane anymore.

I think my un-diagnosis is probably inaccurate, and the improvement in my condition is due to much less stress in my life. I just keep moving ahead, regardless of what it's called. Life is an adventure. I intend to enjoy it.

So what can we say to Bunny, Tara, Dee, Barb, and all the other folks who have gone through every diagnostic process available and are still not sure what they're supposed to believe about themselves and MS? Somehow it doesn't seem right to say, "I hope you find out that you really do have MS," even if that would be preferable to living in the unknown that Nadiza mentions. On the other hand, saying, "I hope you find out that you don't have MS," sounds like a wish for those people to continue to exist in limbo. I guess it's best to wish them peace in whatever they find out. Peace, and maybe the courage and determination to say, along with Barb, "I just keep moving ahead, regardless of what it's called. Life is an adventure. I intend to enjoy it."

5

The ABCs of Treatment

Helen Isn't it funny how our well-intentioned friends are always looking for a cure for us? One night my phone rang. It was my retired beekeeper friend in northern Wisconsin. He's eighty years old, still very active and health-conscious. He was excited because he'd seen an article about bee stings as an MS treatment. He wanted me to hop in the car and drive up there to use his bees. He even offered me his spare room to stay in while I'm undergoing "treatment." I told him thanks, but that, unless he alerted their emergency services, I wouldn't be able to take him up on his offer, since I'm allergic to bee stings. The poor man was so bummed! He'd thought he was going to be able to cure me.

Dee There are so many reports of "cures" coming out—people go into remission and then think it was this or that thing that caused it. Somebody is always telling me about some other person who was "cured."

Dev A friend of mine called me one night and told me I should be taking lots of evening primrose oil because it would cure MS. I had heard it's good to take if you have MS, but not that it's a cure. I decided I had nothing to lose by trying it. After three days of taking it, I had an attack and landed in the hospital. Needless to say, I'm not cured. I'm still not sure if the primrose oil triggered the attack or if I was going to have one no matter what I did or didn't do. Anyway, my friend says I didn't take it right. Sheesh!

It wasn't long ago that people with MS had to look to those well-intentioned friends, to sensationalistic media reports, to anything that offered hope of relief from the ravages of multiple sclerosis. There wasn't much else available in the way of long-term control of the disease. I remember seeing a segment on a television magazine show once about a woman with advanced MS who was struck by lightning and immediately regained sensation in and use of her whole body. Several people asked me later if it would be possible to voluntarily undergo electric shock in the hope that it would reproduce the effect of the lightning. It was hard to not conclude, right along with them, that it might actually be a good idea.

Now, finally, we can relinquish some of our desperate imaginings. While there still is no cure, we have a variety of new treatments that have been proven and approved to help slow the progression of MS. These are the so-called ABC drugs: Avonex®, Betaseron®, and Copaxone®. As recently as two years ago, when the manuscript for *Women Living with Multiple Sclerosis* was completed, only a few of the ladies in the Froup had tried any of them. In the short time since then, most of us have begun to use one or another of the ABCs.

Our doctors are as grateful for these new, long-term treatments as we are:

Dr. Reed The National Multiple Sclerosis Society (NMSS) announced in 1999 that all patients with newly diagnosed MS should be given the opportunity to participate in immunomodulation treatments [the ABC drugs, as well as other immunosuppressants, work by inhibiting activity of the immune system]. This has made a great difference in the way we treat patients today, compared to the days before 1995. Finally we can say to the newly diagnosed patient [and those not so newly diagnosed] that there is treatment available to slow the progression of the disease. We used to have to tell our patients, "We will treat your symptoms, but there is little we can do to treat the disease itself." That has all changed today. This goes a long way to ease the frustration of both the physicians and the patients.

We'll start with a brief description of the makeup and usage of each ABC drug. Avonex® and Betaseron® are both manufactured using interferons, one of the proteins that occur naturally in the body. Copaxone® contains synthetic polypeptides and naturally occurring amino acids (which make up proteins). All three are administered by self-injection. Avonex® is injected intramuscularly once a week. Betaseron® is injected subcutaneously every other day, and Copaxone® goes under the skin every day.

Those last couple of lines aren't meant to be a cue for "needle-phobics" to turn around and run (okay, I'm speaking figuratively), screaming, "No way could I ever stick a needle in myself!" It is a scary prospect, not so much for fear of pain, but more because the idea of jabbing a needle into one's own body seems unnatural, somehow macabre. I'm one of those who swore I'd never be able to inject myself, and I do it every day now. Virtually all MSers can learn to administer their own medications. Family members are encouraged to learn the procedure as well, so they can take over on days when the patient just can't handle it. For those who absolutely can't or won't do the injections, there's always the possibility of having them administered in the doctor's office or of having a home health care professional administer them.

The comments that follow are excerpted from conversations the Flutterbuds have had about their own experiences with whatever ABC drug each happens to be using. They aren't meant to indicate that we, as a group or as individuals, either endorse or denounce the use of any one medication over another. The decision to use one of the drugs, and the choice of which drug to use, should be made by the MSer together with her doctor. The potential benefits and side effects, the patient's history, and the methods of administration should all be considered before making a decision. Also, keep in mind that the experiences of our ladies may or may not be typically associated with the medications. As with everything else about MS, we have to avoid absolutes when we talk about the drugs used to treat it. We can only say absolutely that no two MSers will react exactly the same to any one treatment.

The resources section in the back of this book gives names and addresses of organizations that provide extensive information on the ABC drugs.

My own ABC saga began when I was selected by lottery to use Betaseron® shortly after it was approved for general use. I breezed through the next year with almost no side effects, no problems with injections, no flare-ups of symptoms, and I felt good the whole time. But, by the end of the year, I seemed to develop a sensitivity to the drug. I began to break out in hives every time I injected. I tried discontinuing its use, then going back to it, but the same thing occurred. So I stopped using it completely. Just that year on Betaseron® gave me a blessed respite from the MS's progression, and I have reason to believe that its benefits continued for some time after I stopped using it.

Dev I have been in the Avonex® study at the Cleveland Clinic since 1991. I had only minor problems all the years I'd been on it, until this year when I had two exacerbations. Before I started Avonex®, I was having problems all the time and was in the hospital twice because of the MS. I don't know where I'd be today without it. I really believe it saved me.

Laura I've been on Avonex® since 1996. The doctor wanted me

on Betaseron®, but I was too scared of what the side effects might do to my lifestyle. I can plan my life around the possible "hangover" or bad reaction from Avonex® once a week, but not every other day, as might have happened with Betaseron®.

Ramia   I was on Avonex® for two years. Toward the end of that time, I had two exacerbations. During the first one, just the thought of getting out of bed and walking four or five steps caused total exhaustion. The second one caused double vision. The doctor thought that I had built up a resistance to the Avonex®, so he switched me to Copaxone®. When he saw me several months later with my cane and my wobbly legs, he hinted that I might want to switch back to Avonex®. I decided to go along with that, since I'd gone steadily downhill during the time I was on Copaxone®. We'll see how Avonex® works this time.

Kathey   At first my neurologist was reluctant to start me on one of the ABCs, because it seemed at the time that MS would follow a very mild course for me. She said that the possible side effects outweighed the potential benefits. Then I had another exacerbation, and we decided that I wasn't going to be in that "benign sensory MS" group we were hoping for. I was wavering between using Avonex® and Copaxone®, but my neurologist encouraged me to go with "A" because, at the time, there weren't MRI-based outcome reports on "C." I have always been terrified of needles, so this was a big deal for me. [This is our Nurse Kathey speaking, the lady who sticks needles into other people every day!] I was on Avonex® for about six months. It became routine after a few weeks, although that long needle gliding toward my body was still scary. I continued to have flare-ups and continued to "progress." Then I started having fevers, which continued every day for two months. I had a full infectious-disease workup, but there was no clue as to what was causing the fevers. I went off Avonex®, and within a week my temperature was back to normal.

I've been on Copaxone® for three months now. I'd had new symptoms every few days or every week for most of the previous year. I haven't had a single new one pop up, or an old one come back, in the past two months. Is it the Copaxone®? Or is it just a trick of the Beast? I don't know, and I don't care. Something is working, so I'm not changing anything! I guess I'm just grateful that there is something available (besides steroids and ACTH) to help. I can't imagine the frustration some of y'all went through years ago when the doctors had to say, "I'm sorry, there's nothing we can do."

Robin I never really considered not using one of the ABC drugs. I wouldn't have wanted to pass up the chance to try to stop this. I figured, what's the worst that could happen? It might do nothing, but it might work.

Right after my diagnosis, my doctor told me that he wanted me on Avonex®. I started it within the month. It wasn't bad as far as side effects: fever, aches, that kind of thing, for the first couple of months. I just took over-the-counter pain relievers for twenty-four hours after I injected. I did find that sticking to a schedule was important. If I varied days or missed my regular time, I was more apt to have side effects.

The problem was, I was still having attacks almost two years later. I switched neurologists when my first one wouldn't even discuss treatment options with me, then switched to Copaxone®. Three months later, I seem stable. Injecting daily doesn't bother me, maybe because I was already used to the injections. Needles don't scare me anymore. Having more progression of multiple sclerosis scares the hell out of me. I've made my choice.

Kathey I think what finally convinced me to use Copaxone® was a conversation I had with one of the TevaMarion [Copaxone's manufacturer] pharmacists. The ingredients of Copaxone® are amino acids and some mannitol (a natural sugar). They're not essentially different from the things we eat or take as supplements. I like the idea of it being a "decoy," of the MouSies eating up the Copaxone® instead of poopin' in my brain. It's generally not absorbed into the rest of the system. The molecules of proteins are too large to be absorbed through capillaries in the subcutaneous tissue. So the medication just sits there and says, "Hey, MouSies! *Eat me!*" (Gotta admire their attitude, if nothing else.)

I started using Copaxone® in 1999, when a severe exacerbation prompted Dr. Reed to encourage me to try whatever means possible to control the Beast. When his assistant (Dr. Reed's, not the Beast's), Rhonda, was making the arrangements, she mentioned that "training" by a nurse was available through the manufacturer. I was confident I could handle it on my own. After all, I'd injected Betaseron® almost two hundred times; how much different could the Copaxone® injections be? I soon found out. I had problems handling the smaller of the two syringes, seeing the markings on the bottles, withdrawing the solutions; and the first dose got under my skin in more ways than one. It stung, more than any other shot I'd ever had. If it hadn't been for Kathey and Robin, I would have fixed myself a big helping of crow, then called Rhonda back and begged for assistance.

Kathey   I think of giving myself the injections as "stabbing the MonSter." The shots are something I personally, actively do to fight, and that thought takes away my fear of the needles. The other thing I do is ice the injection site. I use an ice pack for about two minutes before each Copaxone® shot, and I don't feel a thing.

Robin   With the Copaxone®, icing really helps prevent stinging. Do it before injecting if you want, and definitely for five to ten minutes after. Also, I've complained to Shared Solutions/Teva Marion about the skimpy measure of sterile water they provide and the hoops we have to go through to get it all out. The directions say to inject 1 cc of air into the bottle before withdrawing the water. I inject 2 cc instead, and the air pushes the water into the syringe very easily. The larger syringe is easier to handle than the small one that's provided. So, after you mix the Copaxone®, remove the needle from the large one, replace it with the needle from the small one, and use that to draw up and inject the medication. Experiment with shot locations to find what's most comfortable—you aren't strictly limited to the places suggested in the literature. The important thing is to inject just under the skin, not into muscle. Shared Solutions has a good website, MSWATCH. It's there for Copaxone® users, although it's open to anybody. It includes message boards, community information, mail, etc. It's a nice area.

Me   I'm glad you contacted the manufacturer with your comment about the skimpy saline solution, Robin. I'm afraid I'm going to break the needle trying to get the last bit out of the bottle to make the required cc.

Kathey   I inject 3 cc of air into the vial, then pull the needle nearly all the way out and tilt it sideways as I turn the vial over. I keep the vial tilted the way the needle is facing. I've done thousands (millions?) of shots for other people, and I'm used to drawing up stuff. But it is tough. Maybe the manufacturer includes the small bottles of diluent because, since they don't contain preservatives, there's concern that folks would try to reuse larger bottles and risk infection.

My major gripe is with the big label on the vial. It's very

hard to tell when the medication is mixed. The bottle itself has to be dark; evidently light can harm the medication.

Me I found it's important to aim for the very center of the vial's top when inserting the needle to withdraw the solution. I hit just a smidgen off-center, and it didn't go all the way through the plug. When I tried to press the plunger to inject air into the bottle, the needle popped off. SCARY! I guess on shaky-hands days, I'll have to get Ron to help me hit the right spot.

Also, Robin, thanks for telling me you don't have to follow the site recommendations exactly. I noticed there's only one belly site; that was my favorite place for doing Betaseron® shots. I certainly have more room to vary the sites on my belly than on my arms, and the belly is easier to reach than the butt! I just realized, you can't do belly shots with Avonex®, can you? I guess you'd need a very big needle to hit a muscle there.

Kathey Or a really muscular tummy, which leaves me out totally. Even if you could find a muscle (ahhhhh, the good old days), it wouldn't be large enough to take the medication. Hips, upper arms, and fronts of thighs have the "big muscles" with more circulatory support to absorb the medication as it is supposed to be absorbed.

Me Speaking of upper arms, you know how hard it is to self-inject there, since you can't pinch and shoot at the same time with only one hand? I've figured out how to inject myself in the left arm. I roll up a big towel, stick it under my arm, then push it against the side of my chest. That pushes the flabby part of the arm out enough to keep me from hitting a muscle. I wouldn't try to do that in my right arm, though, with my left hand. I leave that site for a time when Ron is home to do it.

Marge I do all my Avonex® shots in my thighs. I use nine

sites on each thigh, which means I have eighteen weeks before I use the same area again. That allows for a lot of recovery time.

Laura I do my Avonex® shots in the thighs only (my hubby helps). It is a great way to keep track of location. There are four packs in the box. The first pack is the side of the left thigh, the second is the side of the right thigh, the third is the front left, the fourth is the front right.

Robin After six months of doing Avonex® shots in the thighs, they hurt too much. I guess that's when the spasticity must have started, and shooting into the muscles there made the pain and spasms worse. My thighs used to hurt for two or three days after my shot. I switched the shots to my hips and arms; they were fine.

Donna I hadn't observed the connection between increased spasticity in my legs and pain with thigh shots. You're right! I'm not having problems with spasticity now, so the thigh shots aren't as traumatic. But when I first started Copaxone®, my legs were very spastic; I'd have muscle spasms and pain for hours after the injection. Thanks for making the connection, Robin!

What about the MSers who have a definite diagnosis but aren't using one of the ABC drugs? Is there ever a good reason not to "stab the MonSter"? I'm sure that for some, the cost is prohibitive. Without insurance coverage, it runs about $1,000 a month for each of the drugs.

Margo I'm not on any treatment, and it's due more to stubbornness on my doctor's part than to lack of insurance. I had to ask him several times to write a prescription for Avonex®.

Then the insurance company denied approval, and he hasn't done anything to convince them otherwise. He feels that because I'm progressive, the ABCs would not be very effective. Now, listening to you gals, I've just about made up my mind to try Copaxone®. With this doctor, though, it'll be the same story, so I'm looking for another doc. This is the insanity of this disease: to feel my "clock unwinding" day by day and be helpless to do anything about it. To have a doctor who waves off my requests for one of the ABCs..., could it be any more frustrating?

Debby I'm not on any of the ABCs. We don't have insurance, and there is no way we could handle the cost ourselves. It is frightening, because I see the progression. I wonder if, when I do manage to get on one, it will already be too late. Also, I get angry because if I'd been taking one all along, maybe the MS would not have progressed as much so far. Maybe right now I could be more of a wife and mom to my family.

Robin Debby, you should have said something sooner! All three drug companies have programs for those with no or poor insurance. All you have to do is contact them. If you know which you want to try, call your doctor and call the company. They will help!

Kim Right! If you are uninsured, all three companies offer the medications at no cost or at a prorated cost based on your income. Right now I'm getting Avonex® free for a year. All I have to pay is the quarterly shipping cost. The paperwork is simple. You'll have to send a copy of your last year's tax return and complete their application form. It's a piece of cake! They do ask that you let them know if you get insurance coverage, so the free treatment can be made available to somebody else. I'll have to do that when I get my insurance again.

Nadiza I'm not on any medications. The history of my MonSter's effects so far is that it's mild and slow moving.

Because of the possible side effects, I have decided to forgo the treatments until I feel it would be more prudent to risk the side effects of the medications than the effects of the MonSter.

This is definitely a consideration when deciding which ABC drug to use or even whether to use one at all. The interferons, Avonex® and Betaseron®, can both cause flu-like symptoms, depression or anxiety, and discomfort at the injection site. I was very lucky when I was on "B." Except for occasional site tenderness, I felt fine, with no fevers or aches. Since I had a history of clinical depression, I was concerned that it would return with the "B" injections. But I felt almost euphoric during that year, maybe because I was so relieved that the MonSter seemed to be in hibernation as long as I kept that needle handy.

I did have a particular concern about "C" side effects. I'd read that some patients reported occasional chest pain, irregular heartbeat, flushing, and breathlessness associated with the injections. I'd already had problems with arrhythmia, with two bouts of atrial fibrillation severe enough to put me in the hospital. I didn't like the idea of stirring it up again. Dr. Reed told me to check with my cardiologist before making a decision. The cardiologist observed that there was no evidence that Copaxone® caused actual cardiac complications; it appeared to be only a sensory reaction. He said that he could monitor anything suspicious that might show up. So I went ahead with no fear. I did have an episode of chest pain following one injection, about a month after I started on Copaxone®. It resolved within a few minutes, didn't require any further investigation, and hasn't recurred.

Kathey The only side effect that I've had from Copaxone®, and that most folks have, is a lump like a mosquito bite that lasts for two or three days. It only itches some of the time. If it's bothersome, an over-the-counter antihistamine or cortisone cream takes care of it. No matter which medication you're on, I think it helps to consider the side effects (whether flu-like from the interferons or itchy bumps from the Copaxone®) as proof that the medication is working, that it's doing what it's supposed to do. I assume that it is not just making itself known to me through the side effects, but to the MonSter, too.

Between the hope from all the wonderful, successful research going on and the hope that the ABCs already give us, plus our stubborn, will-not-be-beaten attitudes, we are starting to win this battle. Some of us are doing it armed with needles, some with pills, others with faith. We will defeat it. I believe that with all my heart and every itchy, lumpy inch of my body.

Me   That's the way I look at it, Kathey, especially when I wonder about long-term side effects of the ABCs. I've yet to see a report on what those might be. I guess the drugs haven't been used long enough and widely enough to reach any conclusions about what they can do after months or years of use. We just have to hope that the most common long-term effect will be an ability to stay an inch ahead of the MonSter.

Sally   I was on Betaseron® for about a year and a half, but then the flu-like symptoms started getting really bad, worse than they had been at the beginning. I had to stop using it because I was spending all my time feeling too sick to enjoy anything at all. I have considered going on Avonex®, but I still have a psychological block about that because it is also an interferon. I am waiting to see how others react to the Copaxone®. Hopefully I can wait long enough so that the pill version will be ready when I am.

Me   I wonder how there can be an accurate assessment of the good any of the ABCs is doing. I know that sometimes there are observable changes on MRIs, but those don't always correspond to either stabilization or worsening of symptoms. Whether you get better, stay the same, or get worse, how do you know what is from the medication and what was going to happen anyway?

Kim I wonder this every time I give myself the damned shot. I have progressed from remitting/relapsing to secondary progressive while on an ABC. I wonder sometimes what the purpose is!

Me But then we're back to wondering how much the treatment was or was not involved in the change in your status, Tink. Could it be, too, that the fact that you're considered secondary progressive now might actually be a good result of the drug? Maybe what is being interpreted as slow progression is really just a deceleration of the dramatic plunges of remitting/relapsing. If you're beyond the remitting/relapsing stage, there's actually less chance that you'll have an acute attack that will totally devastate you. I had three of those, plus oodles of little ones when I was remitting/relapsing. But the "knock-down" attack I had last month was the first I'd had in the ten years since I moved to secondary progressive. So, if it's a choice between using Copaxone® and going back to slow progression or not using it and being at risk for more attacks like last month's, I'll use it.

I get irked over those MS "type" labels. I think they try to give us false information about ourselves. As we're all finding out, they don't mean much of anything when it comes to predicting what the MS will do from that point on. Look at Jamie—she's been considered progressive almost since the beginning. But she did very well for many years, better than many of us were doing with our remitting/relapsing tags. Then she got whammed with a supersonic relapse. So how can the assignment of a "type" predict what will happen with or without treatment? It should be enough to say, "You have MS. Anything can happen. Treatments might work. Treatments might do nothing. Have a great life."

Kathey The more I think about it, the more I realize that any chronic disease is unpredictable. Even with something like cancer, you don't know if chemotherapy is going to work, or maybe if you don't do anything but hang in for ten years, something else will pop up that will help. Maybe that's where the "advantage" of a progressive label comes in? Slow decline sucks. Slow decline punctuated with horrid relapses sucks more.

I've heard theories that the different types of MS might actually be different diseases. I think of it as just the opposite. It's all one big unpredictable disease. From all I've read, there are just as many folks who start out wham! wham! wham! with exacerbations (primary progressive?) and end up symptom-free for twenty years as there are who start out "benign sensory" or mild remitting/relapsing and end up getting hit with the "big one" and are non-ambulatory within a few years.

The ABCs are purported to reduce exacerbations by about 37 percent. There's no way of knowing if you'd actually be having 37 percent more flares, or 100 percent more, or 60 percent fewer without them.

Blind faith, lots of research and hope.... That's what I'm sticking with for now (well, that and a handy-dandy half-inch 27G needle!).

One more (strictly subjective) observation about Copaxone®: The drug isn't intended to make MS patients better; it's only supposed to slow the progression of the disease. But several of us have noticed that our symptoms have actually improved since we've been using Copaxone®.

Donna For two years, I avoided using one of the ABC drugs, because I have an intense fear of needles. Then I had an attack that scared me more than the needles did. Five months after starting on Copaxone®, my symptoms have lessened to the extent that I'm able to go back to work full-time!

I don't think I'll head back to a full-time job just yet, but I, too, have noticed that my symptoms are less bothersome, or that I'm better able to deal with them. I just feel less "victimized" by the MonSter since I started on Copaxone®. Would that have happened even without the drug? There's no way to know for sure. Could it be a placebo effect? It certainly could be. We all know that a "take-charge" attitude, the thrill that comes with being empowered to do something to fight the MonSter, can have real physical benefits. It doesn't matter; we'll take the improvement, no matter what caused it!

Of course, the old stand-by treatments are still standing by, waiting for whenever we call on them. The most frequently used is a three- or five-day intravenous infusion of steroids, usually prednisone or, less frequently, ACTH, to calm acute exacerbations of symptoms. Several years ago, I said "never again" at the prospect of this brand of therapy, because I hated the side effects (mental confusion—beyond what's normal for me—mood swings, bloating, severe constipation, complete sleeplessness). Last fall, though, when the MonSter went on the warpath, I was desperate enough to try anything. I went with a "milder" course of oral prednisone and once again gave it up sooner than was recommended because of the side effects. But I did recover from that attack quickly and almost completely. Was it because of the steroids I managed to get into my system or because I started on

Copaxone® at about the same time or just because it was going to happen that way? There's no way to know. But I know now that "never say never" holds for MS treatments, too.

▲▲▲

Sharon   I'm still a firm believer in the steroid treatments, because it seems most of the time they help, or at least they did for me. I worry about the time that is said to come when they no longer help. [Steroids sometimes seem to lose their effectiveness after a patient has been treated with them numerous times.] I don't like looking to the future with no treatment available.

Dee   I hear you on this, Shar. I remember how much the steroid drip helped Kat's trigeminal neuralgia. I also remember my neurologist's nurse and the folks at Urgent Care saying that I can't have this treatment anymore because of my reaction to it. I do believe, though, that there are other treatments around the corner that are going to help stop acute attacks. I'll keep that in my mind and thoughts and prayers, for you and all of us and everyone else who has this DD [damned disease].

▲▲▲

We can also still treat many of the individual symptoms of MS as they pop up. We talk about remedies for pain, fatigue, and bladder malfunctions elsewhere in this book. Then there's the good ol' spasticity, which cramps the style of virtually all of us at some time (or some of us all the time!). Most of us take either Baclofen® or Zanaflex® to control spasticity. It might be helpful to share a couple of our adventures with these drugs.

▲▲▲

Vicki   I'd been having shaky-legs problems with the Baclofen®. [One of the side effects is leg weakness.] I decided to cut my dose in half and take it every two hours instead of every four. It sounded like a great idea. Caution! Don't fall asleep between doses if you do it that way! I slept for five hours this afternoon, which meant my half-dose had to get me through about seven hours. Oops! I woke up, managed to get out of bed, and had a leg cramp that hurt like an s.o.b. I had another extensor spasm while Larry was helping me outside. I was afraid to move anything. I could feel all my muscles knotting up. I still can't move my legs quickly without the spasms starting, but I'm catching up on the Baclofen®, so maybe by morning, I'll be back to normal. I won't be trying to wean off again unless I have something to wean onto at the same time. Do not try this at home....

Barb   And I thought you were a trained professional on a closed course, Vickers! I hope you get caught up on Baclofen®, too. Be careful from now on.

Me   I had something like that happen, Vicki, but it was when I was trying to switch back to Baclofen®, after trying Zanaflex® and being too sleepy to function during the day. The morning after I made the change, I had this "incident" where my whole body went into one huge spasm. I couldn't move anything, could hardly even breathe. I was lucky that I'd headed for the bathroom just as it started, because once the whole-body spasm let go, everything let go. I lost control of my bladder and bowels and, at the same time, got hit with an attack of projectile vomiting. I hadn't been the least bit nauseated, so that was a not-so-welcome surprise. After the whole thing was over, I felt weak and shaky and tired, but not sick. Dr. Reed told me later that I should have weaned off the Zanaflex® while gradually reintroducing Baclofen®; he said stopping the Zanaflex® suddenly was too much of a shock. Now I've worked out a routine of taking Baclofen® during the day and a combination of the two drugs at night. That works very well. I can function during the day and sleep at night. Hey! Isn't that what normal people do? What a coup!

Kathey   I have to jump in about the Baclofen® pump here. [Kathey's obviously dreaming—she's going to *jump*?] It's a truly great device. It's implanted surgically near the spine and delivers about one-hundredth of the normal oral dose directly into the spinal canal. Since it doesn't have to go through your whole blood stream to get to the spinal cord, it eliminates the weakness and fatigue that are side effects of oral treatment. I've heard of several people who are pleased with the results. Let's hope it will be perfected soon and be easy for everyone to get, so that none of us will ever again go through these problems with the dosage adjustment of oral antispasticity meds.

Two of our ladies recently had surgery to treat MS-related problems. Here's Sharon's story:

Sharon   During the past couple of years, my dominant left-hand intention tremor, which began shortly after my MS diagnosis, progressed and was given the label "movement disorder." It worked its way up to my elbow, shoulder, neck, and affected my voice. My neurologist told me that only 5 percent of MSers ever get movement disorders similar to mine. It was so bad, I had to sit on my forearm to hold it still. When I walked I had to hold it behind my back. The constant shaking caused even more balance problems and pain in my neck and shoulders. To make matters worse, there was a "mirroring" action, so that when I used my right hand to type or write, my left would move violently. Consequently, I had no use of the limb or for the limb. I was so devastated, I actually asked if amputation was an option.

After several rounds of steroids and other drugs, I was referred to a team of neurosurgeons in the Boston area for a fairly new neurosurgery called deep brain stimulation [in which an electrode is implanted in the brain to control tremors. It is used most often in Parkinson's disease patients]. This team assured me that they could restore 70 percent use to my dominant left hand. All of a sudden, I had hope!

The surgery lasted about six hours, and I had to be awake for four of those. I had to have the surgery done twice, as the electrode implantation slipped the first time.

The second was successful! My recovery time was very fast. Now I'm able to reach out with both arms and take my granddaughter to me! I can stroke my daughter's cheek without injuring her. I can tie my shoes, shave under my arms, write legibly with both hands. I can prepare a meal alone and I can cut my own meat.

I was given the gift of freedom from fear, grief, and loss.

Barb I am so glad you are back to being ambidextrous, Shar.

Sharon Thank you, Barb. It's great to be able to do things like hold open my checkbook, hang up my clothes, hold a piece of paper still while I write on it, stuff an envelope, pull on a pair of pants with two hands, hold my zipper with one hand and pull with the other, hug my husband with two arms.... Shall I go on?

Me Sharon, that's wonderful to hear! Thank God the surgery happened when it did. Can you imagine how frustrated you'd be otherwise?

Sharon I'm just beginning to realize exactly how frustrated I was. Imagining how much more frustrated I might have gotten is a road I don't wish to travel right now. I'm so wrapped up in gratitude, I can't even begin to think about the consequences of not having had the surgery.

I'm so happy to be alive, yes, even with MS!

One success story is heartening; a second one seems like a miracle. Tara's involved surgical correction of a brain malformation (Chiari syndrome) that wasn't directly related to MS, but that had a direct impact on MS for her. She had severe pain in her neck, shoulders, and arms and had lost most of the use of her arms because of limited mobility. At times, it was impossible to tell which of her symptoms were related to the malformation and which came from MS.

Tara   My skull in the back at the bottom was too small, and my brain was squishing out....Ouch! The doctor removed the bottom part of my skull, took a graft from the top of my head, and added it to the dura, the tissue that surrounds the brain. That made the whole thing bigger, so it's no longer squishing my brain. I have done well from that surgery and now have full motion of my neck and arms, with no more headaches!

Later, the surgeon found that I had a syndrome that caused me to have compressed nerves in the wrists, elbows, shoulders, and collarbones. It's much like carpal tunnel syndrome or ulnar and thoracic entrapment, for you medical types that understand that. For those of you who don't (that would include me), let's just say it's a big owie! My physical therapist thinks that this was all caused by a very spastic thoracic spine and that my upper body was already weakened by MS, making it even harder to live with. So more surgery on that!

Shortly after her surgeries, Tara updated us on her quick recovery.

Tara   Well, gang, I am feeling wonderful! My incision gives me some pain, but the fact that I can whine about it means it isn't anything too awful. I get tired a little faster than I did before surgery, but that is just part of the recovery from the procedure and will pass. I'm doing exercises to increase my endurance and the strength in my arms and legs. I don't feel any adverse effects from them so far, just some nice, healthy muscle burn. That is a treat, so I have no complaint on that one!

This is truly an exciting time when it comes to treating multiple sclerosis. There are enough options available now so that at least one will probably be "right" (helpful? manageable? affordable?) for each MSer. Add nutritional supplements, exercise, physical and occupational therapy, meditation, prayer, peer support, and good old common sense in with the drug and surgical treatments, and we have an arsenal of weapons with which to fight the MonSter.

Dr. Reed   There are many therapies that relieve discomforting symptoms. However, there are still many symptoms that cannot be relieved. Here the patient slowly learns, just as the physician has over the years, that some symptoms take some getting used to and just must be endured. The physician must be willing to keep trying. Often, the simplest treatment helps unexpectedly, when one does not really understand why. The old motto of, "Don't just stand there; try something," often works here.

Kathey   I think we should come up with a "Serenity Prayer" for MS treatments.
   God, grant us
   patience to listen to caring folks when they are excitedly telling
us about the latest miracle cure;

faith in medical science when our doctors say, "Here, stick this needle into yourself every day/other day/week";

and the wisdom to know the difference between treatment and snake oil.

Something like that. Once upon a time, penicillin was mold on a piece of cheese in a Petri dish. Who ever would have thought it would turn into a miracle?

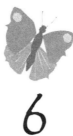

6

The Doctor Is In...Or Out

Kathey Well, Buds, I got home a couple of hours ago from my appointment with the neuro-ophthalmologist whom my neurologist said was "the best." I was in the room with him for less than five minutes. Here's how it went:

Doc: "Well, Miss C., exactly why are you here? What is it that you think I can do for you?"

Me: "Dr. Bremen wanted you to check my eyes. I've had optic neuritis in my right eye for six months, and my left eye is now showing signs of it. I have double vision, other strange distortions in my vision...."

Doc: (rolling eyes) "And what exactly am I supposed to do about that?"

Me: "Dr. Bremen wanted you to evaluate my eyes, to see if you had any suggestions. She is considering starting me on oral steroids for several other MS-related problems I am having, and...."

Doc: "Oh, and I suppose you are going to tell me about that flawed study about oral steroids being bad for ON [optic neuritis]?" (eye roll again)

Me: "Dr. Bremen didn't want me on oral steroids until it was clarified whether or not I had the beginnings of ON in my left...."

Doc: "Well, I can tell you if you do or not, maybe, but I don't see what difference it would make. You're losing your vision. Face it, you have MS." (eye roll and smirk)

I didn't say anything as I grabbed my coat and purse and walked briskly from the office, thankfully not once tripping over anything or running into a wall.

I am so furious! Worst of all, as I walked past the desk, the receptionist called my name. She was filling out my bill—all she had down so far was $110, $78, $52.

As soon as I got home, I left a message on my neurologist's voice mail. Then I called my insurance company. I've spent the last hour collecting addresses (American Academy of Ophthalmology, National Eye Institute, American Medical Association, Health Resources and Services Administration, and the like.). The letter I type, after I calm down, to this "doctor" (quotes intentional), with copies to the insurance company, my neurologist, the National Multiple Sclerosis Society, every hospital where he's on staff, as well as all the above mentioned agencies (plus a few more, as I think of them) will be a masterpiece.

I truly don't know when I've been this angry. This guy is the *best*?! If a clerk at McDonald's treated me this way, I'd still be complaining to the manager two hours later. Oh, I'm so incredibly mad! And I still can't see worth a shit!

Me   Kath, maybe you should suggest in your letter that *he* see an ophthalmologist. I'd be kind of concerned about the way his eyes keep rolling.

Donna   You go, girl! I've dealt with a doctor very similar to this one. I'm glad you know where to write to report this jerk. I didn't, and was afraid to create much of a stir since he was the doctor who was doing my disability examination for my pension. Once again, you go, girl!

It's conversations like that which spur exchanges like this:

Me Donna, this guy was known as Dr. Gotcha Overabarrel?

Donna Either that or Dr. Gonna Makeafortuneoffyou.

Everybody chimes in:
  Dr. I Am Clueless
  Dr. I Can't See Whatajerkwadiam
  Dr. Nota Rocketscientist
  Dr. Ima God
  Dr. Headup Hisass
  Dr. Arrow Gant
  Dr. Dumb Fnork
  Dr. Dip Shit
And the favorite of MSers:
  Dr. Inyer Hed

Dev How about Dr. Gone Again? When I want to see my doctor, I call his travel agent. That guy is never in the United States (but the travel agent gives great medical advice!). I'm supposed to see him later this month. If he's not there, maybe the nurse will have a picture of him. I'm beginning to forget what he looks like.

Margo Okay, you guys, it's my turn. I went to see Dr. Dumbass yesterday (you know, the one I've been going to for nearly three years now). I asked him how his end of the paperwork was going in preparation for starting Avonex®.

He: "What paperwork?"

Me: "The paperwork the insurance company sent you some time ago requesting more information."

He: "Look, I don't play those games with insurance companies. If they want more information, you call them and find out what they want."

I just sat there with my teeth in my mouth. Remember last month, when he was so enthusiastic to get me started on Avonex®? After that, I could not believe this. Can *anyone*

believe that a person with MS would have to fight this hard to start a treatment? It's been seventeen months since I was officially diagnosed, and this is the shit I've been listening to for all this time. I didn't dare tell him that I'd been thinking about going on Copaxone® instead.

So today I got a letter from my insurance company that says, in effect, that since the doctor hasn't replied to the request for more information in the last sixty days, the company is discontinuing action until Dr. Dumbass follows through. Never mind, because I am *never* going back there.

By the way, this guy's waiting room is always full, while, across the way, another neurologist's (the one with whom I'm making an appointment) is empty. That has always made me nervous, like, "What's wrong with *that* guy?" But I've decided maybe he's the smarter one, that perhaps he doesn't cram nineteen hundred patients into a day. I've just been too damned loyal to Dr. Dumbass for the past three years. Well, fuck loyalty! I'm out of there!

Me Margo, if I were you, I'd follow your decision with a letter to the doctor you're dumping, telling him exactly why you're dumping him. I can almost guarantee you won't get an answer, but at least it will make you feel like you alerted him to his own stupidity. Good luck with the new guy!

Helen I think you also should turn him in to the American Medical Association and to the insurance companies, especially the one that wants information from him. Call them and tell them he's a bungling asshole (not in so many words, perhaps) and that you will find another doctor who will take care of the paperwork. What a ratbastard!

Kim This might warrant a call to the state department that regulates MDs. He is at fault, and his actions are jeopardizing your condition, because he "doesn't play the insurance game."

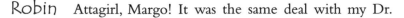

Robin Attagirl, Margo! It was the same deal with my Dr.

Asshole. He was so nice to me in the beginning, and then, because I didn't take his word that all I needed to do was dope myself up four times a day, he couldn't be bothered with me. On my last visit, I was treated downright shabbily. So don't you dare go back there! Obviously, he doesn't care about his patients. That's probably why his waiting room is so full—he's entertaining himself jerking off in the bathroom after every patient he sees. He probably has wet dreams about intertwining nerves or something.

I'm sorry this happened to you, Kiddo. I think I'm finished now.

At this point, I know that not *everybody* is finished—I'm sure there are other horror stories to relate. But I have to pause in our discussion and make a disclaimer. We know that not all doctors, and not even many doctors, incite such fury in their patients. I can immediately name a list (and I'm sure the list isn't complete) of Flutterbuds who have only respect and affection for their physicians. Kim, Vicki, Sharon, Joy, and Nadiza have all told us about their doctors, the ones who go out of their way to let patients know that they care about them, rather than just *for* them. It's sad that the pompous asses are the ones we end up talking about most of the time. For many of us, with MS or any other chronic condition, doctors are the hinges of our well-being. We usually end up seeing several on a regular basis. The actions of each are interconnected with those of the others; if we happen to get a rusty hookup with one, the whole chain of care is broken.

I've had my share of rotten docs. My first neurologist diagnosed MS, then tried to convince me that each symptom that subsequently turned up did so only because I'd imagined it. I spent sixteen years denying, at least to myself, that I really had MS. I blame him for all that time spent doubting my own sanity. I also had one primary-care physician who refused to prescribe anything stronger than ibuprofen for fibromyalgia pain. I had an immunologist who, after I'd scratched myself raw from what I later learned was chronic eczema, told me, without even glancing at the affected areas, that I had dry skin and should put lotion on it. I said something like, "This is so bad, sometimes I want to die just to make it stop itching." He said, "That's good! I can give you an antidepressant for that!" So I know firsthand the huge impact that an unsatisfactory doctor/patient relationship has on us.

Margo   It has occurred to me that lately I've been letting depression rule my life. I had given up in almost every area, and, frankly, I think it had a lot to do with Dr. Dumbass, who treated me like just another heifer in the cattle call of patients he sees every day. Tuesday, I'll go to the "other" guy, and, believe me, he's going to get an earful. I want to start on Copaxone® and Provigil®, and I want *him* to do the insurance paperwork he's supposed to do. It just galls me that I've been diagnosed for more than a year and still am not on any of the standard treatments.

Joy   Margo, I understand your impatience and anger. Just remember that honey catches more flies than vinegar. Any doctor tends to get pissed off when a patient marches into the office and demands certain medications. Docs have this crazy idea that *they* are the experts and should make those decisions. So just go about your requests gently, and I'll bet he listens. He'd better! Because, yes, it's time you got decent medical care, and you have a bunch of dangerous women backing you up!

A few days later:

Margo   Well, I finally did it. Yep, I went to the new neurologist today. This guy behaved in a way totally unfamiliar to me, and I'm not sure how to take it. I think Dr. Lahiri actually acted like... a *doctor*! What a concept! He not only wrote the prescription for Copaxone®, but also gave me tips on how to get it at no cost (we'll see about that...). He did hesitate about prescribing Provigil®, though. He says he wants to test to be sure I'm not narcoleptic first.

    This guy even laughed at my jokes! His staff was easygoing, upbeat, and cheerful, unlike the stressed-out, overworked gals at the old doctor's office. The appointment today, including the whole neurological exam, lasted about an hour. And time spent in the waiting room? I didn't even have a chance to read a magazine. Wow! I'm afraid to be hopeful, but I'm so grateful just for getting as far as we did today.

Vicki   He acted like a doctor? Not just an actor that plays one on TV, but a real doctor?! How odd!

    We have more ideas about the qualities that we appreciate (or not!) on the doctor's side of the doctor/patient alliance:

Debby   My first neurologist came into the room and, without a word, proceeded to examine me. Then, he called my husband into the room and asked what made *him* think that I was having problems. He talked right over my head, as if I weren't even in the room. If a doctor needs to ask a question about me, then ask *me*. If he wants my husband's perception of it, then ask him that. Don't treat me like a child who's too stupid to understand the question; make me feel like I have a role in what is happening to *my* body.

Kathey I've been very lucky with doctors so far (except for the eye guy). I have the advantage, too, of my nursing "knowledge" and research abilities. I've been presented a couple of times with a situation where I got incomplete answers from a doctor. In those cases, I just said, "I would like X testing done," or "Tell me what you think of X drug/treatment."

Maybe it's my ego that allows me not to think of doctors as gods, but as the gatekeepers to comprehensive health care. I admire their education and experience and knowledge. But I always remember that I am the "customer" in the doctor's office. None of us would think of walking out of a jewelry store with a $1000 watch without having our questions about it answered and, most certainly, not if what we really wanted was a watch battery.

I never allow a doctor to rush me, either. Being in a super busy office doesn't mean that my problems or concerns are not important. Think of the salesperson analogy again. If you were buying clothes, would you accept the salesperson saying, "That looks okay; take this one; don't ask me why; just believe me; I have ten customers waiting"?

I ask questions. I call and leave messages for my neurologist frequently (she always calls back promptly). The same goes for my primary-care physician (PCP). With my health maintenance plan, I know that my PCP is being paid to oversee my care, whether I ever set foot in his office or not. I do tend to ask questions only when my other research options have been exhausted, so mostly I present them with a theory and ask for the doctor's input as it applies to my care specifically.

I think of doctors as service providers, and I expect good customer service.

Dev This is where I made my big mistake. I always took the doc's word on everything. I just figured he knew more, so who was I to question him? But then I started thinking (scary, huh?) that he doesn't know *me* or how I feel. So now I ask about everything. Of course, now he looks offended because I ask questions. I can't win.

Nadiza   I don't think the majority of doctors are self-serving, heartless bastards. I think that, after a while, many doctors forget that we are not just their "line of work," that there are human beings behind the charts. Some do not realize the indignities that patients go through until they themselves are patients. My own neurologist, although she has been a very caring, thoughtful doctor, who has always treated me as though I'm an intelligent woman, did not quite get the magnitude of some of the difficulties that we have in dealing with life day-to-day, until one of her MS patients died all alone. Then another one of her MS patients who could no longer live alone told her that she would rather die than go into a nursing home. That's when Dr. Prasad gave her second apartment over to this woman and two others with MS. They all improved considerably because they felt like humans again.

Kathey   If I have a leak in my roof, I'll call a roofer and have him come out and take a look and let me know what he thinks needs to be done. Then I'll look up information about roofs. Then I'll call another place for an estimate. Then I'll call the Better Business Bureau to check out the companies who gave the estimates. I'll ask neighbors and friends for recommendations. And that's just for a danged roof! Why don't we care enough about ourselves to give at least that much consideration to our health care?

Instead we say, "Oh, okay," when the doctor says, "You have a flu virus. Take these antibiotics" (catch that irony—virus/antibiotic—umm, that doesn't work). We say, "Oh, all right," when the doctor says, "Well, your tests are negative. Try getting more rest."

Don't get me wrong; I think the whole mysterious aura

is sometimes propagated by the health care industry. We use strange words, make you wear butt-revealing gowns, put you in rooms with bright lights and loud noises, with a bunch of strangers participating in the most intimate of circumstances. Let's face it; if you'd been naked in front of the grocer a billion times, would you still call him "Mr. Smith"? Nope. But how many patients are lucky enough to feel comfortable calling doctors by their given names? We ask patients to become numbers or worse yet, conditions. You know, "the pneumonia in room 153." I wonder who is really served by maintaining the depersonalization and mystery of health care?

The doctors don't even know the patients in the hospital. But, do they listen to our (the nurses') suggestions about what is really going on with a patient? Never (and, yes, I'm comfortable making that blanket statement)!

Kim [also a nurse] I agree in some ways, but I think that, many times, the docs get calls at three in the morning for things that could wait. We had a couple of assholes, but for the most part, the doctors we had were great guys! I guess doctors are just like the rest of us. There are good ones and there are asses. They can't really be lumped together!

I remember hearing, some time later, about the doctor who diagnosed me. We talked on the phone, and then, while I was on the way to see him in the office, he went to his desk and cried. It really bothered him to have to tell me. Maybe it's having to deal with this kind of thing (giving news like, "You have MS") that makes doctors seem distant. Maybe, instead of being assholes, they're just trying to protect themselves from the hurt.

Kathey That's probably true. And we can't always give the doctors all the blame. Just as I know that there are lots of not-so-good docs out there, I'm aware that there are lots of not-so-good nurses, too. I've learned a lot about being a patient in the past year, and it has made a big difference in the kind of nurse that I am. It's so easy to get cynical when you see people every day who seem to just need a swift kick in the pants. Now I know that maybe what they need more is somebody to listen, to understand, and to care about them.

So I try.

Me   I believe you do, Kathey. You've also brought up something that I consider to be a big factor in establishing a good relationship with a doctor. The first impression we have of a doctor usually comes from his staff: the receptionist who answers our calls and the nurse who greets us and prepares us for an examination. My experience has been that, if I feel comfortable with those people, I'll feel comfortable with the doctor, too. I guess their attitudes rub off on each other. Or, maybe caring doctors seek that same quality in the people they hire to assist them. For example, I'd want Dr. Reed as my neurologist even if his nurse were a paroled axe murderess. So, it's a real bonus that the two ladies who work with him, Rhonda and Sandy, are always friendly, compassionate, competent, knowledgeable, and helpful beyond what I'd expect of them.

I truly like and trust all the doctors I see now and their staff members, too. Maybe there are more great doctors out there than we realize. If there are so many crummy ones, how did I end up with all good ones at one time?

Kathey   Something that we should all do is call our local chapters of the National Multiple Sclerosis Society and let them know about our good or bad experiences with different neurologists. They keep a list so that newly diagnosed folks (or anyone) can call and ask for recommendations. That can make it easier for other MSers to end up liking their doctors.

We realize that we have to do our part, too, to make our visits to the doctor go smoothly.

Kim One thing that helps with my visits to Dr. Jung is that I bring a list of the medications I'm on, the doses, and which refills I need. Then I list anything that might have changed in my condition since the last visit, followed by any questions I have. That ensures that we cover anything urgent right away, and it leaves us time to talk to each other about other things. It really works well. Doctor Jung commented that she likes to see an upbeat patient once in a while. It's not that she expects it on every visit; I am certainly not upbeat all the time anyway. But it gives her room to see more of me than just the part that needs medical management.

Me Isn't it neat when a doctor seems to *want* to know more about us as people, Tink? These are the ones who aren't afraid to let us know a little about themselves, too. From what you've told us about Doctor Jung, I'm sure she's like that, and that's why you feel "upbeat" when you see her. Dr. Goodman (my gynecologist, whom I like to call "Dr. Good Man") sometimes chats about everything but medicine when I'm there. He tells me about his new projects or asks about my writing or wants to know how Karen and Julie are doing. Of course, he's also doing the necessary examinations while we're talking. He has spoken lately about the benefits of a holistic approach to medical care. He definitely incorporates that into his practice; I always come away from his office feeling that he has cared for every part of me.

Chris When I see my doctor I always take two 3" x 5" cards. One has all my medication information on it, so we both know which ones I need refills on. The other one has my questions and new things I want to talk about. I would never remember any of this if I didn't do that.

Me I do the same, Chris (if I remember it ahead of time!). But I type my list of medications on a sheet of paper. Lately, in fact, I keep a file in the computer with all the information about my meds on it. It's simple enough to keep it updated when one of my meds changes. Before I go to see a doctor, I print out the latest update to take with me. When the nurse says, "What medications are you taking now?" I hand her the paper, and she can insert it in my chart without writing everything out.

Joy I read just yesterday that many HMOs expect doctors to limit their average routine office visit time with each patient to ten minutes! Speed is part of the efficiency now demanded to keep health care costs down. I think we can do our part by being prepared (with our lists) to make the best use of the time the doctor spends with us. I guess we'd better restrict our jokes to one-liners, huh?

Tara I call my primary-care doctor immediately after seeing a specialist and ask the nursing staff to let him know that I had this or that test, it showed such-and-such, and I'm starting physical therapy for it or having surgery or whatever. The next time I see him, he is already informed about what's been happening, and he doesn't feel left out of the loop.

Joy You've made some important points, Tara. In the team approach to patient care, one doctor—the PCP, usually—should oversee everything, coordinate the care. Doctor B., my last PCP, was quick to recognize when I needed a specialist, and he kept tabs on which were the most competent specialists available. So when he referred me to someone, I knew I was in good hands. But the system doesn't always work perfectly. Dr. B. never received the radiologist's report from my last set of MRIs, for example. Your method of follow-up would be an effective way of keeping your primary-care doctor informed.

I asked Dr. Reed for his thoughts on what we, as patients, can do to establish and maintain good doctor/patient relationships. Typically, he hands much of the responsibility back to the doctor:

Dr. Reed Patients must be *patient* with their doctors, and doctors must be willing to listen, explain, and try new things with patients. Caring for patients with a chronic disease takes a particular type of physician. There are those who need the instant gratification of making their patients well with quick procedures (i.e., surgery). These are the ones that may not have the endurance to get through the tough times with the MS person. Those caring for the chronically ill often burn out at an early stage. Burnout does not necessarily mean these doctors will quit, but they may not be the most understanding physicians. Doctors are human and suffer the same maladies others do in professional roles. It helps to have a staff capable of easing the load of the many patient calls every day. Experienced personnel who can answer many of the questions and do much of the counseling in a compassionate manner are invaluable in our practice. By sharing the burden, all can carry on longer and support each other. [See what I mean, Rhonda and Sandy?]

Then there are the understanding, considerate patients that really make our day.... Most patients fall into this category. They are supportive of us and often sense when we are having a bad day. These are the ones we appreciate, the ones that make our work worthwhile.

Thank you, Dr. Reed, for not saying that an MS patient can ruin her relationship with her neurologist by bugging him to write something for her book!

7
The Worst of the Worst

Pick any symptom or sign of multiple sclerosis, and it's bound to be the one that several members of our Froup claim to hate the most. Pick another one five minutes later, and those same ladies will say that one is the worst. They're all awful, so it's hard to decide which wins the prize. But certain ones crop up repeatedly in our conversations as being the biggest challenge. Virtually all MSers experience these, at least occasionally. So we can talk just briefly here about what is wrong and why it's wrong. Then we can move into sharing the ways we've come up with to make pain, heat intolerance, fatigue, cognitive malfunctions, and loss of bladder and bowel control less "worst" for us all.

Dee I've always had pain, and I thought that was mostly from fibromyalgia. I don't know, though. I am fifty-five, and I often wonder what part is MS, what's fibro, and what's just plain age. Sleeping is one of my biggest bugaboos. I'm trying to sleep in bed as opposed to the recliner, but I get very sore in bed.

Me Dee, can you check into getting an adjustable bed? I slept sitting up on the love seat for more than a year before I got mine. I can't sleep in a completely reclining position; that causes too much pressure on trigger points. That much of the pain is from fibromyalgia, I'm sure. But there's also pain from spasticity in my legs, and that's probably from MS. Getting an adjustable bed was the best thing I could have done for myself. I have a kind of routine now. I usually start out semi-sitting, which keeps my neck, shoulders, and back from pressing into the pillow or mattress. If my legs go into spasm, I raise the foot of the bed. I can get through most of the night like that before the pressure on my hips gets painful. Then I lower the head and feet for the rest of the night. It took some time to figure out the rotation of positions that was most helpful. Now I dread not being at home to sleep in my own bed for even one night.

Vicki Would insurance cover the cost of an adjustable bed?

Me It would depend on your policy, Vicki. Mine would have covered part (probably about half, after co-pays and a required rental period) of the cost if we'd bought it through their provider. But the provider sold strictly hospital beds, and the price started at $2,000 for a single-size. Ron and I went to a regular bedding store and paid just a bit more than that for two singles. We put them together to make a king-sized bed that looks like (is!) a real bed. It ended up not costing any more than if the insurance had helped. Since Dr. Bennett, my primary-care doctor, had prescribed it for me, half of our total cost qualified as a medical deduction on our taxes.

Dee I have thought about looking into that, and that's what we may eventually have to do. The same thing happens to me if I lie flat. It creates too much pressure on certain trigger points. A waterbed used to be very comfortable for me—but that was before MS. I'm wondering if it would be too warm now?

Me We had one for about fifteen years, Dee, and yes, I had to keep the heat turned way down (enough to make it actually too cold to be comfortable for sleeping) or I'd wake up numb and weak and dizzy. On the other hand, since water at room temperature feels very cold on your body, lying on the unheated waterbed was a great way to stay cool on hot nights.

Helen I have a very soft futon over a mattress and, over that, a soft pad. It keeps the pressure off the points and still gives me support. I find that a soft surface is what I need, like a "feather bed" sort of thing. Since I am allergic to feathers, I made a pad of cotton lined with quilt batting. When I am having a lot of pain, it comes out of the closet and goes under the softest sheets I own.

As it turned out, Dee didn't have a chance to make different sleeping arrangements before the pain took over in every area of her life. She ended up going, reluctantly, to a pain clinic for help. However, she found that her reluctance was unwarranted.

Dee The pain clinic was great! I'd been dreading it. In the back of my mind I was thinking that the staff there would want to take my pain medications away and replace them with biofeedback or something like that. This was not the case. I was there for about five hours and saw a psychologist, a medical doctor, a physical therapist, and a pharmacist specializing in pain.

They believe that the long-acting oxycodone that I take really does help my quality of life, and I shouldn't worry about becoming addicted to it. They say addiction is a legal term, not a medical one. When you take a narcotic because you are controlling pain, it is completely different from taking illegal drugs or using legal drugs illegally. Yes, I could get dependent on it—but there is nothing wrong with that. When I want or need to go off of it, it will be by gradually tapering off. The pharmacist said that I shouldn't let society make me feel that I'm doing something wrong by taking these drugs, because I *need* them. It took a huge load off of me to hear that. I no longer feel the need to apologize because I am taking narcotic pain medication. My body needs it, and that's the way it is. If that can change, great; if not, I am happy that I have the medication.

There are other areas that I'm to work on: exercise/swimming/walking (little by little); keeping a journal about how I feel to see if I can find patterns to my pain; and pacing, pacing, pacing.... I'm also to discipline myself to care for *me*. I'm to make sure that each day I set times to exercise, write in my journal, meditate—to do what *I* need first and then work everything else in around that! This is a totally new concept for me. I've always ignored my needs until everybody else's were taken care of.

It was an eye-opening day for me, and I would recommend it for anybody who needs help with pain.

Barb   Dee, I want to know about pacing. You made all the other points so clear, I'm sure you can explain this and help us, too.

Dee   The way that the doctor explained pacing to me was very different from how I was trying to do it. I'd thought I was "pacing" by spreading out the things I had to do instead of doing them all in one day. As it was, I might start by taking Mom to the doctor and to the store. Then I'd come home and do my regular things, but nothing major. The next day I might go to the doctor myself and then run some errands. The third day I'd end up not doing anything, because I would be beat from the previous two days. If, in between, something outside my control happened which took up a day or two, then I was primed for a flare-up of fibromyalgia and/or MS.

The doctor told me that I need to exercise, meditate, eat, socialize, do relaxation exercises, first, for the sake of my health. Then I can add the other stuff if I'm able and want to. He said this would avoid using my good days to do as much as possible, then crashing and burning. It will create a more balanced schedule and help to prevent "overdoing." When I told him that I would have a hard time saying, "I can't do that because that is my exercise time," he replied that I don't need to explain why it has to be that way. He said it's like financial advisers telling you to "pay yourself first." I'm trying it, and it does make me feel less frustrated about never having time for myself. And my guilt over the pain medications has dissipated.

I've never felt guilty because I need narcotic pain medicines. But the rest of the recommendations that Dee gathered at the pain clinic would definitely be helpful to all of us. It's especially hard for people with conditions like MS to give ourselves permission to do something for *us*, before trying to take care of others around us. I depend so much on Ron and my girls and other family members and friends; if I'm able to do something for them at any time, I feel I have to make that my first priority. I, for one, will keep Dee's lessons in mind and try to implement them.

The suggestion about keeping a "pain journal" might be especially beneficial. I don't pay enough attention to the things that cause undue pressure on sensitive areas or that send my muscles into spasms. Prior to the start of one recent pain flare-up, I'd been spending most of my days at the computer, doing work that required changing discs every few minutes. I noticed that each night my left leg was painfully spastic and my hip hurt worse than usual. Then I realized that when I reached down and to the left to change discs, the action forced me to press my hip into the chair and my foot onto the floor to keep my balance. Ron moved my computer tower to the top of my desk, and the pain and spasms disappeared. I believe I'll become aware of other pain triggers if I remember and track what I was doing just before the pain started or got worse.

Me   Dee, the plan sounds like it would work for improving a lot of physical problems. Do you think it's aimed at more than just pain; I mean, could it actually help to control other MS symptoms?

Dee   Yes, I think so, to some extent. The theory is that the better you feel, the better your general health is, the less chance there is that you'll have symptoms. I think this has more to do with fibro than MS, but I would think it could help both. Although I'm not sure if anything (except maybe the ABC drugs) really helps to keep MS exacerbations away, we all know that stress and fatigue make the symptoms worse, no matter what illness we're talking about. It can't hurt to be in good general health—as much as you can anyway.

From spring through fall every year, pain takes a back seat to our problems with heat intolerance. For us, it's not just a matter of being uncomfortably hot; the MonSter thrives on heat and attacks with a vengeance when our body temperatures go up for any reason.

Bren   I used to be a real sun worshiper. Now I'm basically housebound from May until September. I go from the house with air conditioning (AC), to the car with AC, to a store with AC, back to the car, then to the house again. If I go outside, it's usually at night. If I'm not in a swimming pool or lake during the day, forget it. I'm in an air-conditioned house.

Heaven forbid that any of us lose our air conditioning! It's not a luxury for us now; it's a basic necessity of life.

Donna Our air conditioning has been broken. The heat breaks me, too. It kicks up all the MS stuff, and it makes me drowsy, but it's too hot to sleep. We finally got it fixed today. It feels wonderful! The job was finished at 4:47 this afternoon—not that I was watching the clock or hurrying the guys along at all. I'm proud that I didn't wear out the cattle prods keeping the guys on task. All I can say is it's a good thing guys can pee standing up. There would have been hell to pay if one of them had had to poop after the promised time to get the AC up and running. I wouldn't let them sit down that long and I'd have been very angry if they'd messed up my carpets. But they got it finished. I immediately turned it way down and took a nap.

Now Gary is complaining about having to wear his hunting coat to watch TV. His fingers are too numb to punch the buttons on the remote, so I get to watch what I want! I'm winning all the way around!

Kim I'm so glad to hear that you got it up and running without a lot of shit on your carpets, Donna. Hope you enjoyed that cool nap of yours (bitch!).

Margo My best suggestion, if you have to be out of the air conditioning, is *wear a hat*. I am a former letter carrier, and where we live, it regularly gets well over 100 degrees. Here are a few ways I used to survive summer: as I said, wear a hat; put a wet whatever (scarf; kerchief; cooling, silicon-filled bandana) around your neck; if you're going to be out for a while (as in traveling), take an ice chest, along with a wash-cloth in a zippered plastic bag. You can soak the cloth in the ice water and put it on your face and on your "pressure points" (neck, wrists, back of knees); keep a dry towel handy, too; rehydrate yourself (no alcohol or caffeine); snack on grapes or other juicy fruits—this helps you rehydrate without adding too much to the bladder misadventures; put baby powder in your shoes, your underwear, anyplace you can manage that makes you feel cooler.

It sounds like a lot of work and a lot of baggage to tote around. But believe me, I am very heat sensitive and have several years' experience in this department. I've learned that it is well worth the inconvenience if it prevents heat exhaustion, heat stroke, or worsening of MS symptoms.

A note to "maturing" women MSers: I've heard from three doctors that the hot flashes of menopause can cause problems with MS. I know that every time I got hit with one, it left me too weak to move at all until I cooled down and recovered. So if you have to grow older with the MonSter (shudder!), do it without hot flashes. At the first sign of "the change," see your gynecologist to set up a program to beat the heat (hormone replacement therapy and/or use of vitamin E, several herbal supplements, and soy products might all help).

Nadiza   The thing I would most like to overcome is the fatigue. I think that is the most misunderstood symptom that we face. Other people have no concept of the overwhelming fatigue that we feel. They do not understand that doing very simple things can bring on indescribable tiredness in a short time. They think that merely exercising our bodies into shape would make us less tired.

Joy   I phoned my doctor's office today and left a message asking his opinion of the new drug Provigil®, which I've heard helps fatigue for some MS patients. His assistant called back and said no one there knew anything about it; she was going to contact the pharmacy for information. I phoned the pharmacy later to ask if any prescriptions had been phoned in for me, and I mentioned Provigil®. The pharmacist said that it is for narcolepsy, but they don't stock it. Does anybody know anything about this?

Helen Provigil® is meant to treat narcolepsy and has been found to have beneficial effects for MS fatigue in some cases. Ramia and Kathey take it and are reporting good results. I'm going to ask my neurologist about it tomorrow, since fatigue is getting the upper hand with me.

Bren I take Provigil®, when I can get it. It costs about $200 a month. But it seems to help tremendously without affecting my sleep. I've tried several other meds for fatigue. They either didn't do a thing for me or actually made me sleepy!

Kathey I think the Provigil® helps me with everything. Because it makes me less fatigued, I have a lot less cognitive crap, and that means two fewer things that I have to deal with. If I don't take it, I feel as if I haven't slept for two or three days; my mind is whirring on nothing and flitting around from thing to thing; my whole body is achy and stiff and uncooperative; my frustration tolerance is low; my reasoning skills are zip; I have no short-term memory and very little long-term, either.

It's like living in a carnival house of horrors combined with a house of mirrors. Look at that, look at this, where am I? Where should I go? Where is the door? Where are my keys? Where was I supposed to go? Where am I now? When am I supposed to leave? Look over there, where am I? Who am I? What am I doing here?

With the Provigil®, I'm at least functional. I mean, I can sleep (and do, a lot), but I can also think. Yeah, I'm still on the Provigil® bandwagon.

I don't take any medication for fatigue; I didn't like the side effects of the one I used for more than a year. But I've been using one little trick (besides taking my "have-to-have nap") that really helps to avoid fatigue. I budget some "bonus" time into my schedule. For example, if I think that fixing dinner will take an hour, I start working on it ninety minutes before I want to put it on the table. Then I can grab a half-hour break while something simmers. I also make it a point to stop working on any ongoing project before fatigue catches up with me. If I'm already tired when I stop for a break, then I dread going back to it and reliving the tiredness. If I stay just a few minutes ahead of burning out, I can rest for a while or switch tasks, then go back to whatever I was doing with enthusiasm.

Some of us think the worst thing we experience is sensory overload, accompanied by serious mental "flutters."

Kathey For me, sensory overload, too many things assaulting my senses at once, and cognitive "foggies" go hand-in-hand. I can't think right even when I'm totally alone; put me in a situation where there are sights and sounds and people and movement, and I just shut down. I think this is the MS symptom I can trace back the farthest. I used to be such a social person, but slowly I withdrew from all my friends, from all my social obligations. Family get-togethers, which used to bring me such joy, turned into stress-filled hours with horrid panic attacks that sent me running to the car to leave as quickly as possible.

I spend a lot of time alone. Josh stays in his room, not out of adolescent independence, but simply because he knows that for some reason (I hope he truly understands it isn't because of lack of love on my part) I would rather be alone.

I think this is the one thing that our families must really

resent and not understand. How can you understand when someone says to you, "I love you with all my heart. Now please leave me alone. No, don't just sit with me. No, I don't want to talk. No, I don't want to go to the movies. No I don't want to eat dinner with you. Leave me *alone!*"?

Vicki Luckily, my family does understand. When everybody was here for Christmas, my mom told them not to stay long. She even wanted to have the gathering at her house so I could leave if I needed to. She knows I can't stand crowds anymore. It's not the people that bother me, but the noise and confusion that come with the people.

Kathey I don't get into this cognitive fog or the sensory overload at work. Maybe I feel a deep sense of responsibility for my patients, and that overrides it. But why don't I feel that for my own son?

My contact with y'all on the computer is on my terms. I can read as much or as little e-mail as I want; I can answer when/if I feel like it. It doesn't take the place of "real life" contact, but without it I'd be totally isolated. I can't force myself to go out and have fun, because it simply is not fun to go out. The cognitive fog and the fatigue make it difficult, if not impossible, for me to live life as part of the world, instead of as a bystander.

Me Is locking yourself in your room twenty-four hours a day the only solution to sensory overload? Has anybody come up with something more practical?

Bunny That's my solution, JL. I hide in a room, close the door, and make the world go away. I hate being in crowds, hate the stores, hate being where a lot of people are. Even when we have the kids on our "Kid Weekends" (don't you just love split homes? Not!), sometimes they drive me nuts. I have to go into my computer room and close the door, or

I'll explode. I don't want to take it out on the kids. After all, it's not their fault. I've even found that I like my time alone after Paul goes to work. So, the only solution I have when I get that way is, yes, locking myself in a room. I'm hoping someone else has a better answer to deal with this!

Me   That's okay, Bunny. It *is* a good answer. The other day, when I was working (*not* playing!) on the computer, Ron and Julie came in to talk to me, one after the other. I did my instant transformation into MaBitch, screamed at them, one after the other, to leave me alone. After we mended all the bruised feelings, we decided that, from now on, I'll do exactly what you said (close the office door) when I don't want them to bother me. Sometimes it's the only way to avoid a triple murder/suicide.

Donna   I've tried everything I can think of to distract myself from too much noise and activity. The only thing I can do is remove myself from it. A nap helps, but most of the time I'm too keyed up to sleep. There have been times that I've become so affected by the sensory overload that I've developed vertigo. Those are the times that I've had to take a tranquilizer and go to bed. Once things have settled down and the world has stopped spinning with every movement, I'm fine.

Debby   I've found one solution for sensory overload is to do something distracting physically. For example, if I'm sitting in church (and our meetings are very noisy, with almost two hundred little children), and it gets so bad it's like my head and skin are buzzing, I pinch my finger or rub my wrist. It somehow lessens the overload of sounds and movement, kind of short-circuits it.

As Kathey mentioned, sensory overload is often part of, or brings on bouts of, cognitive difficulties. Sometimes it's the "flutters" we recounted in detail in *Women Living with Multiple Sclerosis*. Those aren't too hard to deal with, as long as they're not dangerous. Those flutters, which were responsible for us getting to know each other on the Mental Flutters message board on America Online, and which were the source of our Froup's name, are usually light-hearted little brain farts. They make us confuse tomatoes with tornadoes, Republicans with raccoons. They cause our perception of the sights and sounds around us to be slightly off-kilter. They make us read the label on a package in the freezer as "rustproofing sauce" instead of "roast beef in sauce." They make us lose our way as we travel from bedroom to bathroom. They make us forget our own kids' names. Most of the time, if we just stay calm, they're more funny than infuriating. I think they exist simply to remind us that even this MonSter is laughable at times.

It's different when our minds seem to blank out completely. We can't comprehend what we see or hear; our thoughts go in circles without arriving at any conclusions. As much as we like to joke about our flutters, *this* kind of mental malfunction isn't funny; it's frustrating, disheartening, and scary. It helps to understand what's happening in our heads and to have a store of commonsense tactics to get through those times.

Kathey I want my mind back. I've always prided myself on my intelligence, my intuition, my brain. Now I can't remember where I put my car keys. When I find them, I've forgotten what I was going to use them for. I can't remember what the word for keys is a lot of the time.

Sally Kathey, don't panic. I can say "me, too" about the cognitive stuff. I have been dealing with it for several years, and I think I have a handle on some of it. When I am out of my normal routine, I get the cog tizzies. I think extraneous stuff, anything beyond what we normally deal with, requires more mental processing. We have to analyze the situation and decide on reactions. When we are in our normal routine, we have already done each thing before, so we don't have to think much about what we're doing. People without MS or other brain problems get tizzied out over new or unusual happenings, too. We notice it more in ourselves because we are working closer to the bone. We don't have as much leeway for utilizing our mental capabilities, because what would normally be reserve mind power is used up on all the other things that bug us. Sometimes the MS doesn't let us have access to adequate mind power to begin with, much less allowing a reserve. The average person just brushes little mental lapses ("flutters") off to lack of sleep or being in love or whatever is going on at the time. Instead, we are afraid of losing what little we have left of our minds, so we notice it more.

I find it helps to calm down, take a breath, relax a minute. Then go back and begin again to do what I was doing, only more slowly. The more I dwell on "am I losing my mind?" the more scared I get and the less I can perform the chore. As an NMSS peer counselor, I have talked with some folks who have severe cognitive problems. Believe me, I have not seen evidence that you are anywhere near that point (any more than the average person is). So relax, and rest assured, when the chips are down and you have to react the right way, you will.

Me   Does anybody else have strategies for dealing with all of this, besides papering the house with Post-it® notes?

Chris   I have Post-it® notes all over the place!!! But they don't help in conversations or TV shows and movies. What about when I'm part of a conversation with my friends and can't remember what we're talking about? I feel like a total idiot! I can't watch a stupid half-hour TV show without asking

Mike, "Who's who and what's going on????" Yellow notes don't help with those things. I usually just say, "It's the MS!!!" What else is there?!!!!!

Kathey I try to laugh about it. You know, the kind of laughter that is sharply edged with irony? Cleaning up the house helps; chaos is made worse by a chaotic environment. A place for everything and everything in its place—okay, so I'm working on it!

Me That does help me, Kathey. It goes back to what Sally said about our problems worsening when we get out of our routines. For me, "routine" means putting things back in a set place all the time. If I keep my house in order (even if it isn't clean all the time), I can think of something I need to get, go right to the place it's supposed to be and get it, before I forget what it was I wanted and why I wanted it.

Kathey Prioritizing is important, too, assuming you can remember what is truly your highest priority. I make a lot of lists, print up lots of stuff I find on the Internet. Organization and prioritization. Is "prioritization" a word?

Me I couldn't find it in the dictionary, Kathey. But we'll let it stand. We know what you mean, and if you come up with something we can understand at first glance, even if it isn't a word, we'll take it!

Helen Lists. I make lots of lists. And sometimes I even remember where I left them.

Me I bet that sometimes you can even read what you wrote on them.

Dev That's me! I made one the other day, and I didn't know what the hell it said. So much for remembering.

Debby I've had to force myself to be more organized and aware. For instance, I was always losing the receipts to our debit card. Since it comes right out of the checking account, that can create a real problem with balancing the checkbook. Now, every time there is a receipt or I do something by phone, I write it in the register and file the receipt in my wallet. I have to be aware that I have no choice but to do this every single time. I also keep a calendar and a schedule book. If I have something scheduled, I always ask the person I am doing it with to remind me ahead of time. I find that the worry about forgetting something important often causes me to forget more, so taking that extra step to remove the worry helps a lot. I have also found that if I repeat several times, out loud, what I am trying to remember, it somehow gets set in my head better.

Me   I keep a date book in my waist pack, a schedule book by the phone, a memo calendar on the kitchen wall, and another calendar in my office. I often go to social things with my sister Joyce and to appointments with my friend Donna. I count on them to remind me. So one of them calls and says, "Aren't we supposed to go to such-and-such soon?" And I say, "Umm, let me check my calendar—after I figure out which one I wrote it on."

Kim   I have one of those little tape recorders that stays with me everywhere. If I need to remember something, I just tape it. Dad is now asking me to record things he needs to remember, too.

Judging by the input from the ladies, I've had to conclude that I've saved the worst for last: bladder and bowel control problems. Only a few of the ladies' narratives of "accidents" are included here. But we could all change the times, places, and circumstances for each and tell it as one of our own.

Dev I have an appointment later this month to get a bladder scan. A week ago I was having all kinds of problems peeing, but for the last four days everything is back to normal. I don't get it. The doctor said I didn't have a bladder infection. Now it's like I never had any problems. Oh well, I'm just happy everything is working.

Tara When I am very well rested, my bladder acts normally, too. When I've been physically active, my muscles spasm and it takes five minutes to start at all. Then it starts and stops and starts and stops. I self-cath only as I need to, but the doctor wants me to do so three times a day.

Dev This is what I've been experiencing, too. I can't go, but when I finally do, it starts and stops. When it happens during the night, it keeps me awake. I've been sleeping regular hours for the last week and haven't been doing a lot of running around, and it's much better. I never thought of rest as a factor, but it makes sense. I'm not sure what I should do.

Me Dev, one word: *catheterize*. It covers a multitude of sins and prevents another multitude. It sounds horrible right now, I know. But, believe me, someday you'll want to kiss your catheter. (Rinse it off first, okay?)

Dev I know I should, Lynn, catheterize, I mean. I'm wrestling with myself on this one. What if I couldn't do it?

Me Unless your hands are really numb, you shouldn't have any problem, Dev. Check with your doc to see if he can refer you to somebody who can help you learn. My first primary-care doctor sent a nurse to the house to teach me, and it was a very easy experience. Once I learned the basics, my urologist told me I could skip all the "sterile" procedure. Now I just cath, with no sterile prep, and reuse the catheter with a rinse after each use and a cleaning with antibacterial soap once a day. It's really simple, Dev, and immeasurably helpful!

I've also seen a self-cath "helper" advertised. It's a shield that has an opening that, once the shield is in place, guides the catheter directly into the urethra. The ad says you can't miss the right place when you use one. I'm hoping that none of us ever has to resort to something like this, but it's nice to know it's available, just in case.

Kathey Dev, please keep the appointment with your urologist. I did the same thing recently, and I'm glad I did. Here's how my urologist appointment went. First, he asked for a clean-catch urine sample (the kind where you wipe off, pee some in the toilet, then pee in the cup). Then he did an ultrasound scan of my bladder to see how much residual there was (how much pee was left in my bladder after voiding normally). Then he did an exam, pretty much like a pelvic. He also did this thing that somehow measures the nerve impulses "down there." I thought it was going to hurt, but it didn't.

The doctor concluded that I had what is called "door-handle syndrome." I'm basically okay, except that when I realize it's time to go, if I don't get to the potty fast enough, or undo my pants fast enough, *uh-oh!* Soggy drawers.

There's a sphincter at the outlet of your bladder and another one at the urethra (the outside "opening"). My outside one doesn't hold as well as it should, and the internal one lets go too early. The doc prescribed Detrol®. It's like a miracle!

Robin I have to agree. I've been taking Detrol® lately, and it has helped a lot. I still get the *urgent!* warning sometimes, but it eases after a bit. It's not like "I gotta get to the bathroom *now*, dammit!" It's more realistic, like "Maybe I *should* go to the bathroom." I definitely notice the difference when I don't take it.

Me I'm off the Detrol®, Robin, at least for a while. It worked wonders for a few months; then it just quit working at all. I guess I developed too much of a tolerance for it. I'm hoping that if I stay off it for a while, it will work again the next time I try it. I've gone through a *lot* of diapers lately.

Robin With the Detrol®, along with paying very close attention to how my "BnB" (Bladder 'n Butt) is doing, I've adapted well to the bladder control problems. For me, now, it's really an ego thing. It's demoralizing to use diapers, especially when you have a little one who is just out of them.

Kim I don't mind using them, but I abhor having to buy them. I guess it's like guys going in and buying tampons for their girlfriends/wives.

Margo Can't you order them through the mail? I heard they are much less expensive that way, and they arrive in a plain brown wrapper, so the cute UPS guy doesn't know what he's leaving on your porch. I always figured I'll go that way when the time comes to buy in bulk.

Kathey I'm lucky that I don't have "floods" very often, so I buy just regular thin maxipads. I wear one all the time, to catch any dribbles when I'm rushing to get uncovered and sit down on the potty before it starts. They're a lot cheaper than the incontinence pads and a lot more comfortable. I tested them, and they'll hold close to a fourth of a cup without leaking. I get the kind with "wings" for extra security.

Dev I'd need extra security. I hate the thought that it might go through my clothes. I can't go anywhere unless there's a bathroom nearby. I mean really close.

Me I worried about that all the time, too. I thought of testing the incontinence pads, as Kathey did with the maxipads, by pouring quarter-cups of water into them to see how much they hold. But that doesn't take into consideration how they're positioned in your panties; you know, are they in the right place to avoid leaks? So one day I tested one while I was wearing it. When I got the "too late" signal, I just let it go without even trying to get to the john. It didn't leak a bit! That was just with a pad, so now when I have a "diaper day," I feel confident that it will work without leaking.

Nadiza I can just imagine you saying, "Testing, one, two, pee; testing."

Dev Thanks for telling us that, Judy Lynn. I wear pads all the time when I go out. There are times you can't just leave and go to the bathroom (like when you're standing in a checkout line). So I really needed to hear that I'm safe if my bladder lets go.

Kathey Believe it or not, *not* being able to go is as bad as not being able to stop it. If you don't empty completely, tell your doctor. There are medications that might help that, too. And of course, there's self-cathing, which can help to empty the bladder all the way. If you're dribbling [or gushing!] some, but not emptying all the way, your bladder sphincter probably isn't closing all the way. So bacteria can "swim up" and set up a party with all the residual pee. Not good!

One important thing to remember if you're always worried about accidents: don't do the "logical" thing and limit fluid intake. That will clog up your bowels, too.

Kim This discussion reminded me of a song Steve was singing to me the other night: "You're a Yankee Doodle spastic; You wear panties lined in plastic."

That's *bad*, Kim. Steve would have a grand time making up a song for the next discussion.

Lori You want a good poopie story? How about being at a real fancy Christmas party at Caesar's Palace and completely losing control of your bowels? I did! But, being the stubborn and obnoxious soul that I am, I recovered completely. I was on the way to the bathroom when it hit—I felt it coming on—so, I made it to the stall, took off the fancy little underthingy I had bought for the occasion, threw it away, cleaned myself up and went right back to the party with no one the wiser (except Steve). There were tears while I was in the stall, but I didn't let it get me down for long. I enjoyed myself anyway, and didn't let It win!

Nadiza Now I have to tell you about my disaster, or about my disaster and my solution. *Gross alert!* Today Joe wanted to get me out of the house for a while. We went to the archery range. We got there, and Joe and Allyson started shooting. Suddenly I got the "urge." I walked hurriedly to the bathroom, trying to hold my cheeks together and talking to myself: "I'm gonna make it, I'm almost there." I had several "little" accidents before I got to the building, a bigger one as I was trying to open the door, and a couple more trying to find the light. I had a pad on, which kept it from running down my legs. But it did nothing else. I was a mess up to my waist. I cleaned up the best I could under the circumstances. The biggest indignity was that I had to pull my pants back up, and it felt gross. What a horrible thing for an adult to experience! I wanted clean, dry underwear. I wanted not to smell. I wanted a shower. Those things were all unavailable, so I had no choice but to pull the pants up. I left the bathroom, thinking I'd tell Joe that I would run home to clean up. But he and Allyson met me on the road. It had gotten too cold for them to keep shooting. I had to sit on Joe's seat with my soaked-through, shitty pants. I got home and immediately removed my clothes and got into the shower. What a relief!

Joe told me we should stay home until I was feeling better. I told Joe that I was feeling fine. My lack of control was due to the MS, and it would happen again sometime, but I refuse to be held hostage by the MonSter.

Now the solution: I intend to get some Baby Wipes® to take with me when I go out. I also decided to get some bed pads and put them in a plastic zipper bag with a complete change of clothes to keep in the car. I never again want to ride home in the mess I did today. It was an affront to my dignity as a human being. So I will be as prepared as I possibly can. It won't eliminate the problem, but at least I will have a little more dignity by being able to clean up better.

We went for another drive to an antique mall nearby. I bought an awesome book; you know how much I love old books! This one had a cover that caught my attention. It's embossed in gold, with a picture of Jesus in the center and scenes from his life around his picture. The copyright is 1890. It cost *six dollars*. I was supremely happy that I did not let the MonSter control my day; otherwise, I would not have found this wonderful book.

Robin I'm so glad for you. What a good attitude! I guess I'll get there someday, but after one incident like that, I basically fell apart. It took me the rest of the day to pull myself back together. I hate this fucking disease!

Nadiza I'm not fond of it either, but I look at it this way: I have one chance at life (with this body, anyway). I'll be damned if I'll let some stupid disease get in the way of my enjoyment of it! It may make things difficult, but dagnabbit, it won't get me down!

▲▲▲

Nadiza, you forgot to mention that you carry a lot of courage in your plastic zipper bag. Good for you! And good for us that you shared your experience and your spirit with us! Inspired by your attitude (and that of Lori and anybody else who has told us about similar happenings), one of our "worsts," at least, can be less so.

8
Housework Helps

Vicki Larry and the kids were doing some cleaning today. His family is coming in for a visit, so that explains all the effort. You should have seen them work! We have pitched ceilings in the den and bedroom. Larry even cleaned the beam and ceiling fans with the vacuum cleaner. Then, trying as hard as he could to keep a straight face, he said that he couldn't understand why I couldn't do this during the day while I'm home doing nothing. All I would have to do is balance on a bar stool, hold the vacuum canister in one hand, clean with the vacuum wand in the other hand, looking up at the ceiling all the while. I saw no problem with any of this, of course.

I may need to rest today. Watching all this work has worn me out.

Vicki has come up with the ideal solution to one of the biggest problems we women MSers face as our symptoms worsen: housework! Not all of us have our own versions of Larry and the kids, so the responsibility still falls mostly to us. With limited strength and mobility, diminished energy reserves, restricted arm and hand coordination, doing the chores around our houses can be difficult at best, impossible at less-than-best. Even on days when we might have the motivation to accomplish some housekeeping task or other, we can't always get our bodies to cooperate. They're too busy tripping over, falling onto, knocking down, dropping, or just refusing to move to pay attention to such frivolous concerns as a messy house. Until, as in Vicki's case, the in-laws (or some other dignitaries) plan a visit. Then we might go into emergency mode and follow Vicki's example to commandeer whatever troops are available to do either a fast spruce-up or a marathon "polish and purify," as the occasion demands. At those times, we might vow to keep up with the housework on a more consistent basis.

That's when we're likely to discover that we have to change our housekeeping routines and methods, along with our standards, to be able to keep up with everything. We've shared some of the tricks and tips we've devised for keeping our houses presentable:

Joy Who says my house is presentable? If I don't claim it, I don't have to live up to it.

Me That's what I mean about changing standards, Joy. I used to live as though I was expecting guests every day; my house had to be at least surface-clean all the time. Now it doesn't bother me a bit if the doorbell rings, and I realize I haven't dusted for more than a week. It doesn't seem to bother the guests, either. So far, not a single one has asked where I keep the furniture polish.

Kathey I agree 100 percent with the plaque I have in my kitchen: "This house is clean enough to be healthy, but dirty enough to be happy."

I can't keep it clean all the time, with all the fur and feathers and wood chips and seed and stuff from our critters, so I don't worry about it. Oh, well, at least I did get it picked up and vacuumed last week, and I have to tell you I feel better about it now than I did before. Now to just keep it that way.

Sharon   I have four teenagers and a saintly husband to take care of the house, although sometimes it's more work to keep *them* working than it would be to do it myself. So far my house is presentable, at least according to my definition of the term.

Dee   My secret to easier housekeeping? I have a long talk with my hubby. That usually works.

Me   Gee, Dee, I must be doing something wrong. Sometimes I sit and talk with Ron for hours. I get up and look around the house and it's still a mess!

Dee   You've got to cry and stamp your feet, too! For gosh sakes, Judy Lynn, do we have to explain everything to you?

Me   The crying I could manage, but stamp my feet? If I'd do that, somebody might accuse me of having enough energy to push around a vacuum cleaner or a broom!

But we have to get serious here, or we'll never get the housework finished. The truth is, when my body cooperates, I don't mind cleaning at all (and I realize that I have to run, duck, or hide every time I say that). I don't know if it's a point of pride with me to still be able to do most of my own housekeeping or if I'm just plain obstinate. There have been times, especially recently, when I've had to consider hiring somebody to take over at least the heavier work. So far, though, I've been able to modify my strategies to accommodate the latest declines in my physical abilities. I've even found that cleaning or straightening or organizing can be helpful in getting my body going again. If I've spent most of the day at the computer or the sewing machine, or if I've just been disgustingly lazy, I crave physical activity. The handiest way to satisfy that craving is to dig into whatever needs to be done around the house. It energizes me. I can't imagine having somebody else do my housework. To be honest, I don't even like Ron or my kids to help with it.

▲▲▲

Kathey I can't imagine having somebody do my housework either, even me! I can dream about it, but that's it. I think that's just laziness on my part or setting priorities. Keeping my house clean isn't at the top of my list!

Me Laziness or not, top-of-the-list priority or not, we all eventually have to deal with keeping our houses clean. Have all of you come up with personal tricks or tips to help you get the job finished?

Bren I don't have many tricks, but I'd have to say that the best advice is to simplify, simplify, simplify! Get rid of all the extra crud in the house. Put knickknacks behind glass, such as in a curio cabinet, so they don't have to be dusted so often. Get rid of all old papers, old clothes, old furniture, old dishes, and the like. Keep only what you need. Here's an emergency measure: mark one large box "don't feel like cleaning up," and when you need to have the house straightened quickly, shove everything that's cluttering up the house into that box. Go through it later, or when the box gets full, and decide then what to do with all of it.

Bunny This is a real problem for me. My husband is a pack rat and there's so much stuff in this house. There's no way I can get through the clutter to clean anything!

Joy Bunny, you've brought up a key point for me when it comes to housecleaning. Clutter. I know that several of us are "collectors" and others are simply pack rats (and/or married to pack rats). We could handle housekeeping much more easily if we were "minimalists" when it comes to decor. The more objects in a room, the more work is required to clean that room. But disposing of clutter can be hard: you have to decide what to do with each object. Do I toss it out? Sell it? Give it away? Keep it? And if so, keep it where? That requires a great deal of energy, both physical and mental, and the old MS fatigue and cognitive mess-ups limit my ability to tackle such chores and to complete them once I've started. I can handle the daily "must do" tasks—dishes, laundry, caring for the pets—but the big projects are overwhelming. I look at the huge piles of mixed paperwork and old mail residing on our dining table, and I think that tomorrow I will deal with all of that. Then, when I finish organizing that, I'll start on my office. Then the closets, the garage, the attic. Once the entire house is neatly organized, it will be much easier to keep clean.

So that's my plan for tomorrow. Today, I'm just too dang tired.

Me   I always have to think very carefully about what to keep and what to discard. As soon as I throw away something I haven't used in five years, I need it. If I sell something at a yard sale for a dollar just to get rid of it, I'll find out it's worth big money. I get rid of something and realize right after I get rid of it that it should have sentimental value. So I end up keeping almost everything, just to be safe.

That doesn't solve our problem, does it? I'm different from you, though, in that I love to tackle big jobs, more than keeping up with the everyday things. I guess that's because I can focus on one thing for as long as it takes, without letting myself get distracted by other things that I should be doing. And then I can see a big difference when I'm finished.

Joy   I feel the same, actually. I always have preferred the challenge of a big project. Only in the last year or so has this become a problem, and it isn't that I don't want to tackle the biggies; it's just that I can't.

Margo   I mentioned earlier that I collect teacups. I've

thought about remodeling the entire kitchen, so I can have a custom-built china buffet to display them in. Hey, what's wrong with that idea? It's like Bren said about putting things in curio cabinets. I mean, if they're inside something, it means less dusting, right? But getting rid of stuff? That never entered my mind.

Kathey But there's truth in what you're saying, Margo. You see, no matter how much I have lost of "me," I can look around and see the things I love. I have pictures everywhere, carousel horses, mementos of trips, etc. Yep, it's clutter, but somewhere in all that junk is me.

I think we're back to setting standards for keeping our houses clean. For some of us, clutter is just another bunch of obstacles to get around and clean around. For others, the objects we've collected speak of who we are, and they're more important to us than perfectly polished tabletops.

Karon I don't clean much anymore; I got a housekeeper when the going got tough. But back in the days when I did clean, I remember "stacking the deck" before I began, so that I could operate under the best possible conditions. The night before, I would lay out any tools I needed (cloths, vacuum cleaner, cleaning products) so I didn't waste energy doing that the next morning (I don't recommend this for those of you who have little kids who might wander during the night and get into the things you've set out). Physical exertion (as in cleaning!) makes me hot, which makes me weak. So, when I was ready to start, I'd turn on fans throughout the house, lower the temperature on the air conditioning, pour myself a cold drink, and put on one of those migraine cold packs that are like headbands. Then I'd turn on music everywhere and take lots of breaks whenever I felt the least big fatigued. Given my dear husband's work schedule, I was usually alone, so there was no one to tell me I was lazy or to criticize me for resting when I needed to.

Tara My answer to the housework dilemma is, as many of you know...*homemaker, homemaker, homemaker!!!!!!!!* Thaaattt's all, folks!

Me Thanks, Tara. That was easy, wasn't it?

Tara It sure was! I have to say, though, that people who need help with housework should check with the adult services division of their human services office, welfare office, or wherever else they might be receiving other services. If you don't ask, they may not offer the information that these services are available. I don't have to pay for the help I receive.

My homemaker comes in twice a week. She cleans the countertops, does the laundry, changes the sheets, cleans the floors, runs the vacuum, and does the bathroom. I also get companion services twice a week; my companion does some meal preparation, helps me keep the fridge cleaned out, does dishes, and takes care of other small jobs around the house.

These very special people don't just work on my house; they keep me company and have become my buddies. I don't know what I would do without them. They help me keep my sanity.

As long as I have these helpers to keep up the housework, I don't get worn out from that. I'm sure that if I tried to do it, I would find myself flat on my back very quickly.

Joy This is my problem: there's too much to do, but not enough of me to go around. My budget can only stretch so far, and there are no freebies available around here. In that respect, you are so fortunate, Tara. I'm sure I'm not the only one who envies you for your household help. However, if it meant taking all of the physical problems you have along with the help, I'll keep my dirty house, thank you very much.

Ramia We can't afford daily help, but we've hired a weekly cleaning service. The kids must clean up after themselves, put their own toys away, and keep their own rooms tidy.

Robin Housekeeping tricks numbers one through two-hundred-and-then-some: hire a cleaning service, especially if you are still working outside your home. I no longer have the energy it takes to keep up with everyday family stuff, housework, and a full-time job, too. Julie, my helper, comes in every other week. She's been a godsend to me. Is she perfect? No, but nobody is. She's a demon in the kitchen and bathroom and reasonably good with the rest of the house. It's such a relief not to have to worry about that. My biggest problem now is the day before she comes, when it's up to me to get my family to pick up their crap. I have no qualms whatsoever about having someone else do my heavier cleaning. Given my limited energy, it makes life a lot easier.

Bren Help with housework? Well, ummmm, I have my Al, and I have my children. That pretty much covers everything, doesn't it?

Seriously, I just keep on top of it as best I can. My house is cluttered, far from spotless. I wish I could get it organized and clean and keep it that way. But I don't think it's in my nature, or maybe it's against my religion.

My kiddies do help out a lot. Their main chore is to do the dishes, and they have to put away their own laundry, take care of their own rooms, and pitch in with whatever else I ask them to do.

Chris Lynn, I just do one chore every day instead of trying to get it all done in a day or two (like I used to do!). I have Mike help me with dishes and with changing the sheets on the bed and doing heavy things.

Ramia Bed making—am I supposed to do that every day? I just straighten the sheets and throw the comforter over the top. I can't tuck anything in because the king-size mattress is too heavy for me to lift.

Me Changing the sheets on the bed used to be one of my most time-consuming chores. It seemed like it took forever to straighten the sheets on one side, tuck them in, walk around to the other side, straighten and tuck them in there, then repeat all the walking around and straightening and tucking in for each additional layer. Now I do one side of the bed at a time. I put on the clean sheets, add the blanket, then put on the bedspread, get it all arranged and tucked in on one side. Then I go to the other side, pull each layer into place, tuck again there, and all I have left to do is toss the pillows into place.

Kim Lynn, it helps me to have a schedule of everything I need to do to keep up with the housework. I got one of those daily planners and I keep my "to-do list" on it. Each day that I don't get a scheduled job done, I add it to the next day. I have started a rotating schedule, like Chris. Do this on Monday and that on Tuesday. Of course, my "not done" list is always much longer than my "done" list!

But I think that when I stick to the list, it helps with both the fatigue and the short attention span. I set a kitchen timer for a certain amount of time, usually fifteen minutes or so, then do one thing on the list during that time. I try to alternate a hard chore with one that is physically relaxing. I might, for instance, work on my website until the timer goes off, then go scrub the shower. That way, I get frequent rest breaks, and I don't get bored doing one thing for too long a time. Also, each time I go somewhere in the house, like from the computer to my room, I pick up a few things to take with me and make sure I put them away. I have to confess, there are always a few things to put away—I am a perpetual slob.

Tara I make lists, too. Here's one of my lists of chores I might have to do in a day:

1. Tell Jake to go grocery shopping;
2. Tell him forty-two times, "No, I'm not going with you!"
3. Tell my homemaker what needs to be done today;
4. Tell Jake to just go to the store; damn it, I said I'm not going!
5. Tell my homemaker that, no, the grocery store is not a good place to meet eligible men;
6. Tell Mike to mow the lawn;
7. Tell my homemaker that, yes, I took the dog out, and, no, I didn't meet any eligible men while I was out there;
8. Call my sister and ask her to stop by with some coffee because I ran out of it;
9. Tell my homemaker that, no, my sister doesn't know any eligible men....

Back to serious tips and tricks:

Karon I distinctly remember sitting on my butt to clean the floors, back when I used to clean the floors.

Tara If my feet don't stick to the floor, and I don't step in any puddles, I figure there's no need to clean it.

Me Believe it or not, after the MS made it impossible for me to stand and wield a mop or a broom, I discovered that I *like* to clean floors. At one point during a "weak spell," I was restless, bored out of my mind, and sick of the scum in my kitchen. So I asked one of my girls to get a bucket of cleaning water and some rags for me, then, like Karon, I just scooted around on my rear end, cleaning as I went. It felt so good to move around and do something constructive! Since it's something I can do no matter how I feel, keeping my floors clean is now one of my passions!

Margo Me too, Judy Lynn! If my floors are clean, I feel like my house is clean, no matter what the reality of the situation is. My bare floors are fairly small and easy to tend to. Like you, I do them on my hands and knees (or butt), simply because (a) it's actually easier on my body, and (b) I just feel that they get cleaner that way. Vacuuming is a different story. I'm as anal about the carpeted floors as the bare ones, but since my sweeper weighs about 917 pounds, I don't use it as often as I should. But, yeah, floors are my "thing."

Me We got rid of the problem of having to drag a heavy sweeper around when we got rid of most of the carpets. Now I just run a dust mop over the wood floors, or if I'm having trouble getting around, a dust rag, and use the dirt buster on the area rugs. We did put new carpet in the bedroom, but it's a low-pile berber, in a kind of tweedy design that doesn't show the dirt. It's easy to clean with the little handheld sweeper.

I figure my house is even cleaner now that I can't use the big sweeper very often. When I'm right down there on the floor, working on it with a rag or the dirt buster, I can even keep track of dust on the baseboards and give them a quick sweep with a rag, too. I hardly ever thought to do that when I was standing up to clean and couldn't see what was really down there!

Bunny We're slowly doing the same thing, getting rid of the carpets. We're on the road again to putting hardwood floors down. It's good to hear that uncarpeted floors are easy to keep clean! Yippee!

I have to add here that this whole process of discovering that I like keeping my floors clean was one of my first lessons in living beyond the effects of multiple sclerosis. I found out that every time I say, in effect, to the MonSter, "Okay, knock me onto the floor if you want to. I'll just clean it while I'm down there," I'm handed a bonus. When Ron and I removed most of our carpet, we discovered that there was oak hardwood underneath. It needed some TLC, but we could see that the flooring was still basically beautiful. I started thinking that if I was able to work on floors and actually enjoyed doing it, maybe I could find a way to restore the wood's beauty. So Ron moved furniture and bought me a supply of sandpaper and refinishing products, and I got busy. For the next three months (off and on, but mostly on), I sat on the floors in the living room, hallway, and office. I sanded, scrubbed, stained, and sealed every inch of the wood in those areas. In my not-so-humble opinion, I not only restored the wood's good looks, but actually added to its beauty. My floors have a charming old/worn appeal now, but are permanently shiny and safe from environmental disasters. To top it all off, Ron and I saved several thousand dollars we'd figured it would cost to go with our initial plan to cover the wood with laminate "fake-wood" flooring! Thank you, Mr. MonSter!

Now it's time to do the laundry!

Karon Well, my stepson used to leave his dirty clothes on the floor. So I told him that any clothes I found on the floor would go into the trash can. At the time he was just visiting us, and his suitcase was very light on his trip home! The next time he came, no clothes ended up on the floor (or in the trash can) at all.

Tara I bet his mother really loves you!

Karon I guess his mother made him pay for the replacements. But it worked, didn't it?

Ramia Anything that goes into the wash inside out gets folded or hung that way after it's washed. I am serious about this as far as my hubby is concerned. I expect my son, Brian, to at least be a bit more helpful about it, too. Haley is actually the most responsible one in the family. She always puts her dirty clothes in the laundry room, sorts dark clothes with dark clothes, and so on. She does her best and then some, far beyond what you'd expect from a four-year-old!

Vicki On a good day, I might manage to wash a load of clothes. I might even get it dried. My family has learned to get their clean things from the floor when they want to get dressed. The clothes might get folded, but not often do they get put away.

Kim You are supposed to put them away?

Vicki I've heard that some people do. Some even do it as soon as the clothes are washed and dried. I don't do it that way. I can't imagine not having an obstacle course to go through to get from point A to point B in my house. I mean, if it wasn't for the clothes stacked all over the floor, can you imagine how hard our falls would be?

Kim I don't usually get my clean clothes put away, either. I keep them in a laundry basket.

Vicki But doesn't that plastic hurt when you land on it?

Kim Yes, it would hurt to fall on the basket, but that's for the clean clothes. Usually the clothes I fall over are the dirty ones that are on my floor.

Robin One thing that has happened with the MS is that I am much more apt to ask or insist that the kids help more, especially with things like the laundry. They know my legs aren't great, I have a hard time with stairs, and my balance is bad. Since my laundry machines are in the basement, Brandon's job is to carry the wash down. They've all been learning how to sort the clothes, run the machines, fold clothes, the works. I've been working with them both separately and together, so they can no longer use the "I didn't know how" excuse.

I have another whole story to tell here about doing the laundry. My mom worried all the time about how I managed to carry baskets of laundry up and down the basement steps when I could barely get myself up and down. I came up with the idea of stuffing the dirty clothes into an old pillowcase, then I'd toss the pillowcase ahead of me down the basement steps. I'd do the laundry, including folding it, while I was down there, then have somebody else in the family carry the clean clothes back upstairs. That worked for as long as it had to.

When Mom died, Ron and I decided to use my share of her "estate" to make room for a washer and dryer on the first floor of our house. We added a dining nook onto our kitchen and rearranged the appliances and cabinets in the original area to give us the necessary space. I think Mom would have approved, since I no longer have to deal with carrying baskets up and down the steps. In fact, the washer and dryer are so handy, it's as if there's no work at all involved in doing laundry now. The biggest affirmation of our decision was when we totaled up all of our expenses for the renovation. The bill equaled, almost to the dollar, the amount of money Mom had left me! I could almost see her smiling about the (non)coincidence.

Helen My best housework helper is my dishwasher. It hides

the dirty dishes and, once I run it, is a source of clean ones so I don't have to reach way up into the cupboard to get them.

Tara Ah, yes! Here's how I run the dishwasher in our house: "Hey, Mike, do those dishes for me and leave them in the dish drainer so I don't have to reach for them, okay?"

Kim In our household, I'm the dishwasher.

Helen If you break enough, you won't be....

Kim Great idea, Helen!

Helen Just trying to help you out, Kiddo! (But don't let Dad in on this.)

Kim He's clear across the room. There's no way he'll hear about our little plan.

Me I never imagined that I'd want a dishwasher. But now that our kitchen has been remodeled, we have one, and I don't know what I'd do without it. I kind of follow what Helen said about using it as a source for clean dishes. I try to remember to run the dishwasher in the early afternoon. That way the dishes are clean and dry when it's time for supper. I can take the clean dishes from the dishwasher and put many of them right on the table.

Bren But you have to cook if you also want meals to put on the table, right? I think I'm going have to read this book after it's finished to get some ideas from other Buds for that! I'm not a planner. Ninety-nine percent of the time, I end up at Winn-Dixie about an hour after I should have started cooking dinner, looking for something quick and easy.

I have been reading some very interesting information on "once-a-month cooking." That's something I think I could get into, once I can afford to get all the food I need to cook for the whole month. Basically, you buy all you need and plan all your meals, then spend a day or two cooking it all, and then freeze it. When you need it, you pull it out of the freezer, add your "go-withs" and you're all set. As I mentioned, it's something I could embrace totally, or at least the part about cooking once a month instead of every night. That sounds way cool!

Me   I sometimes cook extra portions of whatever entree we're having and then freeze what's left for another meal. The only problem is that I can't tell Ron we're having left-overs. He wouldn't come right out and say it, but I get the feeling he's not crazy about anything that has been heated more than once. I like to do one-pot meals, like soups, that I can just simmer without a lot of tending. I also like quick-fix frozen things and simple sandwiches. When Ron isn't around, I can get by with meatless snacks, mostly raw veggies and fruits, for dinner.

There's one more thing I have to add that's been a great help with all my kitchen chores. When we remodeled the kitchen to make space for our laundry machines, Ron came up with the idea of buying two extra floor cabinets to match the ones we were installing. He put them back-to-back, added rollers on the bottom, and bought a countertop to cover the whole thing. He created an island that's been a terrific step-saver for me. It usually sits right in the middle of the whole kitchen area, equidistant from the table and my assortment of appliances. Since I can't carry pots, pans, dishes, or whatever from stove to table to sink, etc., I can turn from wherever I am, set whatever needs to be carried on the island, then walk (or wheel, depending on how good a day it is) around, pick it up, turn, and set it down wherever it needs to be. Since the island is on rollers, it can be moved in any direction to make extra space when needed at the table for guests or at the stove or sink for "cluttery" jobs. Even small kitchens, with no room for an island, can be made more accessible and efficient by adding a small rolling cart that can transport dishes, pots, and pans from one area to another safely and quickly.

It was close to Thanksgiving when we talked about tips for making cooking chores easier. Nadiza was planning to serve a traditional dinner, and she came up with a solution for not-so-dextrous MSers to handle the big bird.

Nadiza   My double kitchen sinks are too small to wash a large turkey. I used to use the laundry tub (my laundry room is near the kitchen). The problem was that, because of pain in my wrists, I found it difficult to maneuver the turkey around under the faucet. Two years ago I found the perfect solution. The bathtub! I clean the tub and line it with flour-sack towels. I then put the turkey on a large cookie sheet and set the whole thing in the tub. I have one of those shower-heads that is attached to a hose. I take the showerhead down to the level of the turkey and then maneuver the water instead of the turkey. When I'm finished, I take the turkey out on the cookie sheet. Voila! I have a clean turkey in half the time, with less pain to my wrists.

The flour sack towels get rinsed and tossed into the washer. Then I get someone else to scrub the tub to remove the poultry residue.

Bunny   Don't ask me! Cleaning the bathtub and the shower stall are difficult for me. I usually spray the living heck out of them with a disinfectant cleaner and let it sit for a bit. Then I go back and wipe with the sponge after the cleaner has eaten up all the yucky stuff!

Me   Have you tried those shower sprays, the ones you don't have to wipe down ("Just mist and *walk away!*")? They really do work pretty well at controlling soap scum and mildew.

Except that I'm obsessive, so I still do a disinfectant scrub once a week. Dumb!

Dev I like that spray stuff, but I'm afraid I'll forget it's in there and take a bath. I didn't see any warnings on it or anything like "may cause urinary tract infections," and it says it contains no harsh chemicals. It does seem to work really well. Okay, I'm trying to convince myself that it's fine, since I use it anyway!

Kathey Here's a winner! I am on a fall housecleaning binge (the one I should have done last fall). Anyway, I got out the oven cleaner, sprayed it on, closed the oven, and turned it on, just as I always do. I thought to myself, "Wow! This new stuff doesn't smell nearly as bad as the old kind does."

After fifteen minutes, I turned off the oven and looked inside. It was brown instead of the usual white. I then checked the can to be sure that I had the time and temperature right.... Here's a hint for everyone: EasyOFF® is oven cleaner. EasyON® is spray starch.

I now have a dirty, wrinkle-free oven!

Me What were you doing with a can of spray starch in your house, Kathey? Don't tell me you iron, besides cleaning the oven!

Kathey Shhhhhh! Here's my secret: If you wash curtains and then dry them about halfway, spray them with starch, and hang them back on the windows, they dry wrinkle-free and crisp. It works for tablecloths, too. (I can't find my iron; it must be here somewhere....)

As for the oven, it's easy to clean mine, since it's a wall oven and not part of a stove. I don't know if I'd be on my hands and knees scrubbing out that kind. This one is easy, at just the right height for me and easy to reach into. One advantage you have, Judy Lynn, being a vegetarian, is no broiled-meat splatters in the oven.

Me I eat chicken occasionally, Kathey, and have to cook that, but I hardly ever broil it. If Ron wants to eat any kind of dead animal, he usually volunteers to cook it on the gas grill outside. So how do I end up with meat splatters in the oven? I have that kind of broiler that is under the oven, and it does get messy. Let's see, we bought our stove when we moved into this house six years ago, and I cleaned the oven for the first time last week. I don't think I can blame that on MS, though. I wouldn't clean it more often if I didn't have MS.

I'll remember your secret about wrinkle-free curtains. If I don't have any spray starch, do you think oven cleaner would work?

Gee, I don't know what I'd do without the tips that my Buds pass along!

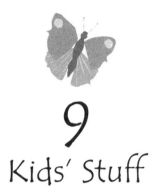

9
Kids' Stuff

SHARON   Bob's oldest daughter, Leslie, is bursting with child, due in July. As Madison's due date gets closer (yes, we know it's a girl), I find myself looking at baby stuff and clipping Huggies® coupons. I also find myself worried about picking her up, holding her, and playing with her. (Sigh.... MS sucks, doesn't it?) I figure that if I get somebody to place her on my lap, I can hold on my knees and maybe feed her that way. But I'm not going to be able to handle her well enough to burp her or change her, because my left hand does not work. Holding onto a baby requires two steady hands. What if my shaking scares her? I don't want my granddaughter to be afraid of her Nana.

My heart goes out to Sharon and to any other women (or men!) with MS who have to fear that their MS symptoms will prevent them from providing adequate care for a young child or grandchild. I was truly blessed that I had only two major exacerbations while Karen and Julie were tiny. During those times (once when I was unable to walk and once when my left arm was paralyzed) I had a whole crew of helpers (Ron, my mom, my four siblings and their spouses, my friends Donna and Phyllis) who almost completely took over the care of my little ones. The next fifteen-or-so years, I was able to mother them pretty well, even when new symptoms showed up. Now I'm in that in-between era, when my girls are on their own and require little, if any, hands-on care from me and my grandbabies are still a fantasy. I don't have to worry about devoting myself to being an always-available, never-tired-or-sick caregiver of kids.

So, for most of this chapter, I'll defer to the ladies in the Froup who have small children or grandchildren. I'll sit back while they talk (and while I wait, not very patiently, for my fantasy to become reality) about the parenting/grandparenting difficulties they encounter and ways they conquer them.

Marge Sharon, I've been there! When we were at Rick's last fall, Jerr had to hand Hailey [Marge's granddaughter] to me while I sat on the couch. That way I didn't worry about dropping her. I wouldn't dream of carrying her across a room. I probably could change a diaper, if Jerr put her on a blanket on the floor, where she couldn't fall. [I almost asked Marge how she'd manage to put the diaper pins in without sticking the baby or herself, until I remembered that mothers now don't use pins—they use self-adhering disposable diapers.] I know what you're going through, because I go through it, too. But I guess I'm just too damned stubborn to give up!

Sharon I won't give up either. Sometimes, though, I want to at least sulk and have a minor pity party. I guess I have reached a point in my life where I know that's a complete waste of time. It doesn't accomplish anything. So now I'll have a pity party because I can't have a pity party!

I'll work around the grandbaby thing when she is born. There have to be ways to do what I want/need to do for her. I just have to start wearing my thinking cap.

Dee With two new grandbabies here, I find it very hard to

accept the fact that I am sometimes too weak even to hold them. The other day when I was at my daughter's, I had to tell her very quickly that I couldn't hold the baby any longer. I started having spasms so badly, I was afraid I would drop him.

We know there are other ways to do these things, holding and feeding, talking, and playing. It's just not the way I'd like to be doing them, the way I fed and held my own kids. I also get the feeling that my children don't ask me to baby-sit very much because of the MS. This actually is kind of them, but it makes me feel even more useless.

I have to break my promise to stay silent here, just for a minute. Dee's comment about not being asked to baby-sit hit home. My niece Tracy has a toddler, Megan, who stole my heart the day Tracy came home from the hospital with her. I've begged to be allowed to baby-sit for her, but Tracy has never asked. That bothered me at first, but as Megan grew, I realized that it would be silly for me to even try. There's no way I could keep up with her. Now I enjoy just holding her on my lap when she allows it. Then, when she gets down to resume her perpetual motion, I watch her. Just watch her. She's the perfect child for an MSer to be in love with. I never have to entertain her. She's an expert when it comes to entertaining herself!

Debby I don't have little babies anymore (my youngest is six now), but I do have little grandbabies. When they visit, I do not pick them up and carry them, even though I ache to do so. If I want to hold the baby, somebody puts him into my arms while I'm sitting down, at the corner of the sofa, so my arm is propped on that and he basically rests against the arm of the sofa.

Bunny I was asked by my friend to watch her newborn

when she goes back to work. She asked me well before she gave birth, and I was already watching her nine-year-old daughter, Rebekah, at the time. I readily agreed without giving it a second thought. In fact, I was ecstatic about it because I never had a baby of my own. After Jonathan was born, I changed my mind on that idea. I've found it very difficult to hold him for any length of time. A few minutes are okay, but then my arms get numb. I'm deathly afraid of actually being alone with him for fear that I'll drop him. Plus, if I'm walking around with him, will my legs go out and we'll both fall?

Wow! These things had never come to mind before. I had to tell my friend that I won't be able to watch Jonathan when she goes back to work, and I explained why. She understands, but it really bothers me.

Nadiza Allyson was eight months old when I was diagnosed. I started out using cloth diapers with Allyson, just as I did ten years earlier with Nicole. But I had already lost some motor control and sensation in my hands, so using diaper pins became increasingly difficult. Faced with either changing my daughter less often (or not at all!) or using disposable diapers, I opted for the disposable ones that taped. They didn't have the diapers with velcro until later. [Thanks, Nadiza. If you didn't have the self-adhering ones either, maybe I didn't do my mothering way back in the Dark Ages.]

Bathing a newborn wasn't much of a problem for me because I had a baby tub that fit on the kitchen sink. The baby only needed minimal support from me because the tub was designed to provide safe support.

Vicki My twins were six months old when I was diagnosed. When they were about eight months old, I lost the use of my whole left side. Try diapering a baby with a useless hand! This was before the disposable diapers had the resealable tapes. [Aha! Vicki is from my generation, too!] I had to redo many diapers that had fallen off. I used up many rolls of masking tape. Luckily, I wasn't working then, so I really didn't have to dress the babies in anything more than a diaper and a shirt. If we went someplace where they had to be fully clothed, Larry dressed them; he usually had to dress me, too!

Kathey I think about that a lot, about how y'all with little kids manage or managed. Even though I'm relatively young (hush up, Bunny!), at least my life is "set" now. I will be more able to fight what the MonSter brings, because I don't have little kids to raise, don't have a new career to start, etc. It scares me to think about it, but, well, I guess this is a "good" time to have MS, with all the promising research going on. (Did I just say this was a good time to have MS? Somebody slap me!) There's a good chance that the people with tiny kids now will stay well enough to raise them.

There's good news to report about Sharon and her granddaughter. Shortly after the baby was born, Sharon had brain surgery to relieve the intense tremor in her left arm. (Sharon told us about the surgery in Chapter 4.) She wrote this a few weeks later:

Sharon Since the surgery, when somebody carries my granddaughter through the door, I'm the first with both arms stretched out to grab her. I can hold her, feed her, schmooze her, nuzzle her with confidence and no fear. *No fear!* What a wonderful gift God has given me!

We know Sharon. She will carry her new fear-free joy past Madison's infancy and through the rest of her childhood. She'll learn as she goes along to make adjustments in her "Nana" role as they become necessary. In the meantime, she can store up the advice of some of the other Flutterbuds.

Tara   I have been trying to watch Ariel in the mornings for Jake when he works all night. It's really not too bad in my house, because she only has access to the living room and kitchen. I put the dog and cat foods up on the counter so that she can't get into them; there isn't a lot of other stuff around that matters. My hospital bed is in the living room, so I put it in a position that is comfy for me, and I lie there and watch her. I talk to her and play with her from the bed. I've taught her how to step on the bottom rung of the bed and climb up when she wants to be there with me. She'll sit on my bed for more than an hour if I keep talking with her. I have to admit that I get silly sometimes and teach her things like "Can you say, 'administrator'?" and "I am the boss!"

Dee   This is so cool, Tara! The way you had Ariel step on the bottom rung of the bed and get up by herself reminded me of when I watch Kyle and Jacob [the children of Terrie, Dee's daughter]. I have taught Kyle to do some things when I am too fatigued to do them for him. He is five now, but since he was three or so, he has learned how to put movies in the VCR, get his own juice, little things like that. Of course, sometimes the only way I can watch the little ones is if Al is there to help. I am lucky that he's always willing. (He is good for other things, too! But we're talking about kids here, aren't we?)

Margo   I've found that I can't do all the "physical" stuff with my grandchildren, but I can do the hugging, the listening, and the "being there" things, like simple craft projects, helping Allie with her preschool workbook, and listening to and exposing her to different varieties of music (as I did with my kids when they were little). These are the blessings of not being able to "wrassle." I honestly think this particular aspect of my life has improved since the MS. I can't work, so I'm home more, which makes me more available. I am weak, so I find myself seeking out simple, special little things we can do together. I am tired, so I often have to use my energy just being a good listener. In this one area, at this moment in time, I'm not sorry I can't be more "physical."

Today Allie asked me to "swing" her; you know, lock my fingers together and swing her back and forth through my legs? Well, you know that wasn't going to happen. So I tickled her and hugged her, and she climbed up on my lap for snuggles. I told her that's what I'm good for: tickles, hugs, and snuggles. I also take her to the library a lot, so we read together, and I always get a children's music CD while we're there. She loves the music and the stories, and it keeps her from wanting to watch TV all day. She has a kazillion other people who can roughhouse with her, so these special times together make me feel "specially special," if you know what I mean.

Dee   This is exactly where I am with my grandchildren, Margo. I have noticed, though, that there is a certain stage of their growth when I almost can't take care of them. They are too heavy to pick up and too young to really pay attention and stop what they are doing. This seems to happen around age ten months to almost two years. At that age, they can get away from me too fast! I always make sure Al is going to be home while they're with me. I can manage the older ones, who are six and eight, because they can take care of themselves for the most part. I can also handle the tiny babies most of the time.

But stairs are a big problem for me anytime. When stairs are involved, I have to sit on them and go down them on my rear while holding the baby. Going up is harder, mostly on my knees. My balance is way off and I'd just die if I dropped one of them.

As they get a bit older, I avoid picking them up by sitting on the floor and letting them crawl into my lap. I do this near the couch, if I can. Then I lift the baby to the couch, and I can stand up by grabbing the couch.

What you said about "being there" as a positive thing is so true. I'd never have known my grandkids so well if I worked full-time. That's why I'm going back to work as soon as I can! (Just kidding, kids!)

Donna The thought that I couldn't do the physical stuff with my grandbabies bothered me badly when I was first diagnosed. At some point, I started to remember my own childhood and the people I felt closest to and why I felt close to them. It wasn't what they did to entertain me that was so great. It was the time they spent with me and the hugs and love they shared that made me feel special. That's what I try to do for my grandkids. And you're right, Margo. Those are the things that make *you* feel "specially special."

Karon My Victoria [Karon's niece, whom she's helping to raise] makes me feel "specially special." She's what I live for! Cupid struck me the day Victoria was born. I really enjoy her, even if she's the reason I fall so much. But she's good for me. I've gotten physically stronger (I guess chasing is good exercise!), and I have more energy (since I can only nap when she does, there isn't much choice) lately. I sit on the floor with her to play and teach. We turn everything into games and learning activities. I love this sponge phase she's going through! I've found out that adrenaline and fear really boost me. For such a shy kid, she certainly loves to experience new things. She'll try anything once! I could go on talking about Victoria forever, but I won't bore y'all with that.

Dee Karon, I'm not bored! I think that what you said about using Victoria's play as her learning is so important. I was often sick when my own kids were growing up, but I managed by doing the same thing. I always think that, just because you can't do things a certain way, that doesn't mean you can't think of a different way to do them.

Debby Sometimes I feel that I've failed my kids because I can't do everything with them. But in some ways, my kids have more of me now than they did before I had MS. I am right here with them, every day, all day long. It's really hard for me to work now, so I'm not "gone." I don't go out with friends a lot like I did, going shopping or whatever. I am here, reading a book with them or listening to how their day went or listening to their corny little jokes over and over. And in the big scheme of things, isn't it the most important thing just to be there for them in whatever way we can?

Dee As you all know, we are visiting our kids and the grand-kids (Taylor is fourteen, Tahni is twelve, and Brady is ten). Tonight they got a new movie to watch. I mentioned to them something about watching it and Taylor said, "Are you going to watch it with us, Grandma?!" They were all excited about it, so Al and I watched it with them. It was a special time together without any walking or physical stuff, just sitting close together on a couch!

Me If I were a kid, Dee, and you were my grandma, I'd be excited about you watching the movie with me, too.

Margo If I was a kid, Dee, and you were my grandma, I bet we'd both be bumping down the stairs on our behinds, using a big, flat piece of cardboard to go faster! Put a little rope on the front end for steering, maybe an air bag for crash land-ings, and, pretty soon, your son and daughter-in-law would be sending you home for too much physical stuff! But the kids would remember it forever. (Does anyone have a hidden camcorder?)

Robin   My bedroom is on the second floor, so all the kids learned to maneuver stairs early. I can't carry them up and down, but I make a game of it, something like "I'm going to catch you if you don't go upstairs," and they race up the steps, giggling madly!

Jenna is learning to be independent. I encourage her to do things like put her wash in the basket when she changes to pajamas. Her shoes go into another basket, which is handy for her to get them out of when she needs them in the morning. I buy her shoes that are easy to put on, too. Kids love to be able to "do it myself!" I tell Jenna what she needs to do and praise her for being a "big girl" when she does something on her own.

All the kids have been taking on more responsibility for themselves and are expected to help out more. I guess that's actually good for them (although they'll disagree!). Maybe they'll grow up to be self-sufficient and independent adults.

Which brings us to another concern that parents with MS usually have. As our kids grow, they might find themselves embarrassed, fearful, or confused by having a parent with MS. How do we help them understand what's going on in our families when the MonSter lives with us, without adding to their fear and confusion? How do we find a middle road between expecting them to take on more responsibility than many other kids their age and compelling them to become preoccupied with trying to make us "better"?

Robin   This part is a little harder to deal with than just finding safe, quiet ways to be with our kids. Danielle is the one who's the most interested in how I'm feeling and asks questions about MS all the time. She helps with my shots or gets my pills for me. She's the one who'll want to give me a hand doing things like helping me up the stairs.

Brandon is the more silent type; he doesn't talk as much about how he feels, but it's in there. One day we were talking about three wishes, and I challenged him to guess what everybody in the family would wish for. When he got to me, he said my first wish would be to not have MS. I thought that was interesting coming from a kid that doesn't usually talk about it.

Jenna is still too little to really understand what MS is. I just tell her that Mom's legs get tired. She won't remember me doing the runaround thing with her or running in a backyard. In a way, it may be easier for her because she's known me no other way.

Brandon and Danielle, on the other hand, did. I'm sure that sometimes they resent me for asking them to do things (like run up or down the stairs for something). But they do it with a minimal amount of fussing, which makes me proud of them. They do understand that I'm not just taking it easy.

Vicki As Ash and Zach got older, when my MS would flare up, I'd explain what was happening, on a level they could understand. The older they got, the more detailed the explanation. Now they even "spread the word" about me. Their close friends watch out for me; they have no problem with pushing my wheelchair or helping me up when I fall.

They don't get too embarrassed anymore. I have had bladder and bowel accidents when I was with them. When that happens in the car, we just hang our heads out the window and laugh. Laughing seems to be the key to making them less embarrassed.

The kids have learned to be more caring for other people, young and old, with physical limitations. They've even gone as far as correcting their peers, if one of them jokes about a handicapped person.

Debby I do not drive as often as I used to, especially when I am having an exacerbation, which makes it hard to do carpools, etc. I've found honesty to be the best help. When I am not feeling well, when I'm shaky or my eyes are acting up, I call the other mothers and they fill in. When I am doing better, we make up for the times when we couldn't do our part.

There have been times when I've had to miss my kids' concerts and other events because I was so fatigued I couldn't get up. It broke my heart, but when the kids came home, they performed for me here, which lets them know that I want to see them in what they are doing.

My biggest help in mothering with MS? I give myself permission to not be perfect. I let myself adjust things according to what kind of day I'm having. When I can't go for walks with Jerry, I lie on the bed and watch him play Nintendo or read with him or play a mean game of Checkers (and for a six-year-old, he's hard to beat! Maybe that's because I keep forgetting what color game piece I have?). I am still involved very much in my kids' lives. On my good days, I try to give them good days; on bad days, we adapt. I've forgiven myself for having to do that. I've also found out that adapting is helping my kids to see different angles of things, too.

Bren When I was diagnosed, Kristy was six and Sarah was four. I immediately explained to them that I had a disease called MS. It might cause me problems, and some of those problems might make me unable to do some things. Maybe I wouldn't always be able to go outside with them in the summer, go to the beach, or physically pick them up. I explained that it was why Mommy had been so tired all the time, and that sometimes we'd just have to have quiet time instead of running around. We could still watch movies and play dolls, and on cooler days in the fall and spring, I'd be able to go outside with them. They seemed to understand. They explained a lot of it to their friends. It didn't seem to bother them very much at that point. It was just a part of their lives and mine.

As they got older, they did seem to be a bit upset or disappointed at times: asking to go to the beach like their friends did, asking me to braid their hair, or wanting me to go outside and play with them. It took a little while, but after a bit, they accepted it all. I always told them I would love to go outside and play with them if I could, but it broke my heart to have to tell them I couldn't. It still does!

When Kevin (Al's son from a previous marriage) came to live with us, I had to explain it all again. He was nine years old at the time. He had never been exposed to anything like MS, and, of course, with me looking "normal," it was hard for him to understand at first. He's come a long way with Sarah's help. I love the way she explains the situation to him. It's as though my MS is something very normal (and I suppose, for her, it is!).

The hardest thing for me to deal with is the guilt I feel at times. Having to refuse to do something for or with them takes a toll on me, especially when I see the disappointment on their faces. I just have to keep remembering that it's the best thing all around, because if I get sick or overdo, then I'll be able to do less with them.

Kathey Josh really was hit hard by my diagnosis. Maybe it's because it's always just been "me and him." The worst part was that I was so self-absorbed for those first few months, I missed his reaction/nonreaction completely. I mean, I was so careful to talk to him, to encourage him to ask anything, and to always answer the best I knew how.

Still, his GPA went from 3.9 to 2.1 in one semester, his room turned into a pigsty, and I found a half-smoked ciga- rette under his bed (I know, big deal, all kids do it, right? But for him, it was a big deal, believe me). I'll never forget, for as long as I live, what he said to me. It was a week or so after I was diagnosed. He was crying so damned hard. He said, "Mom, you aren't going to die are you?" Oh, God, even thinking about it now just makes me shake and cry. He had been holding this inside for over a week, not wanting to upset me more and suffering because I was so upset and weepy that he didn't want to make it worse. So, should I have kept it a secret from him? Should I have not told him? I just don't know.

He has two friends who have parents with MS. Both are in nursing homes. Both are in their early forties. Both are nonambulatory. One has a feeding tube. Both are fairly "gone" mentally. So, do I say, "That won't happen to me, my darling son. You won't ever have to change my diapers. You won't ever have to see me like that," (when under my breath I'm muttering, "Oh, God, please let this be true")?

Aw, crap. I'm sorry. Flutterbuds, I swear I'm not usually this maudlin. I swear that I'm funny and bright and amusing. Just not now.

Tara It is very hard to explain to a child how MS limits one. My oldest son had seen how hard I pushed myself, working a full-time job, then teaching college at night. I remember him saying that if other people would "fight their MS," that they could overcome it, too! Needless to say, he and I had a long talk and I gave him quite a few brochures about MS. In his first year at college, he chose MS as his subject for a term paper. I was pleased to see how he had paid attention and learned over the years!

When he was nineteen or twenty, he talked to me about the times a few years earlier when he'd been embarrassed about me, or "not nice," as he put it. Looking back, he felt awful about it. I tried to tell him that it was part of growing up and it was okay. Not that I would have told him those things when he was that age! At that point I was also over-weight; that and using a cane gave his high school friends ammunition. They'd tell him that it was "all over" for his mom, that she wasn't going to last long, and so on. I guess kids need to be told that it is okay to feel the way they feel; it is what they do about it that matters.

Nadiza Allyson has never known me without MS. She is the most understanding one in the family. She gets the least embarrassed by things like my funny walk. At almost twelve, she is sometimes rather overprotective of me.

I've been through (still go through!) this with my girls. Maybe I should say that they go through it with me. Karen and Julie are adults now, but I know that it has been a hard lesson for them to learn that just because I have MS, they don't have to completely switch roles with me. I talked about this in *Women Living with Multiple Sclerosis* in some detail, including their reactions to having a mom with a chronic disease. Now that they're completely grown (if that ever really happens), I can say that we've had some touchy times. Even recently, they've worried about me to the point that I felt I had to abandon being me and doing what I really wanted to do, just for the sake of relieving their anxiety. (Karen: "Mom, I've decided that we'll skip coming for dinner this weekend, because I don't want you to do anything but rest." Julie: "There will be no taking cabs to the dentist for my mom!") They still want to protect me. But they're now as much my friends as they are my daughters, and I guess most of my friends feel the same way about doing things for me as my kids do.

I've learned, and I think we're all learning more each day, that we have to allow our children's reactions to our MS to mature along with the children themselves. Our kids have to set their own schedules for acceptance, just as we do. It's amazing how differently they react from each other and how their own reactions can change in a short time.

Debby Each of my children reacted differently. My youngest stayed very close to me, like my little protector. He was so worried each time I'd get sick and would ask me if I was going to die. I told him I wasn't planning on dying for a long time, but that we all die sometime, and it is not something to be afraid of. I told him I would always be with him, even if I died. I told him that, if anything ever happened to me, whenever he felt sunshine's warmth, it would be a hug from me. Every time he saw a rainbow, it would be me sending him my love. It sounds corny, but it helped reassure my son (who was five at the time).

My nine-year-old still acts like MS doesn't exist. That is her way of coping. She helps out a lot, but I have noticed that when I am in a bad flare-up, she becomes very hyper and upset. She tries to annoy the other kids and causes little arguments. I think it is her way of trying to make things seem more normal.

My twelve-year-old has gotten protective of me and, at times, angry with me without seeming to know why. She worries much more than the others do.

My oldest daughter at first wanted to know if I was going to die. She was only thirteen when I was diagnosed, right when a young girl needs her mom the most. For some time she seemed nervous to be around me, almost like it was contagious. Eventually, though, she became my biggest helper. She jokes with me when I do something strange, like when I put my frozen pizza into the dishwasher to cook. She also helps me with the housework. She helps me with my hair and personal things when my arm stops working. I am careful to not make her the mom and to make sure she has a lot of opportunities to be a kid. She is doing well with it now. I am trying to show her that, in spite of difficulties physically and cognitively, I will do as much as I can, some days more than others. Also, I try to show that a sense of humor helps a lot.

I've found that being open and honest with the kids has helped the most. Respect their ability to understand and also realize that they are the most afraid of the unknown. If you don't tell them honestly, they will use their imaginations to answer their worries. What they imagine is usually much worse than reality.

Bunny When I told my stepchildren that there was a possibility that I had MS, Jon-Paul didn't have much to say about it; Taralyn asked a few questions. Basically, neither of them had much of a reaction. At least not until some time had passed. Then it was Taralyn who surprised me. One night during dinner, I went into one of my stuttering spells. My friend's daughter was here for dinner. She started mimicking my speech. I didn't take offense, just shook it off as her being a child and not understanding. But Taralyn took offense. She piped right up and said, "That's not funny! She can't help it." I was shocked! And I was very proud of her. Taralyn is almost too understanding. When we go shopping together, the first thing she does when we get inside the store is get me a cart so that I can keep my balance by walking with it. When I tell her that I can't do something with her and start to explain why, she says right away, "That's okay. I understand it's because of your MS." She is becoming quite the young lady at the age of ten!

Kathey As a single mom with an only child, Josh and I have always been close, very close. He's been my rock, my sounding board, my best friend. I've already said that MS hit us hard. It made him have to face my, well, not mortality (although y'all know he was so afraid I was going to die), but I guess my future, my abilities, especially to live independently. He knows that, just as for now I'm all he has, he is all I have. But, looking back, it was really a relief for us both to find out that there was a reason for my mood swings, for my irrationality, for all the things I "just forgot."

I'm so proud of him. I know that in the future, he will continue his advocacy for "disabled people." He is as indignant at folks parking in the "fat butt" places without a placard as I am. He notices things that he really shouldn't have to at his age—hills that are insurmountable in a wheelchair, blocked aisles in stores, lack of accessible parking. He has written several papers for school about MS, so that "people understand more." He is never ashamed to tell people what is going on with me and always is proud of what I can do.

I mourn for his lost innocence, however. No teenage boy should have to know his mom wets her pants sometimes. I worry that he is scared of the future, wondering if I'll need help transferring to a wheelchair or if he will have to bathe me. I reassure him a lot about this, but I know it's on his mind. His friends all know that I can't run him around to places like their parents can (luckily, most of his friends are driving now). He understands when I don't participate in the things other parents do.

He's also had to face the consequences of my cut hours at work. Here he is, seventeen years old, and he doesn't drive. Why? First, because his mom doesn't have the patience to teach him. Second, because I can't afford to get him a car or to pay the insurance to let him drive mine. And, he really can't get a job. I depend on him too much around here.

But things have a way of balancing out. I can't manage to drive him to a concert and then stay awake late to go and get him. So I have to let him go and do things with his friends. I have to let him go.

I'm glad he's older; I'm glad I wasn't diagnosed when he was young. I admire all of you who are raising young kids and can't imagine having the energy for toddlers (whether they be kids or grandkids). At least Josh and I can talk about things; at least he understands (or tries to). He accepts how things are, figures out ways to deal with them, and moves on with life. I hope to get to the place he is sometime very soon.

I had no choice but to tell Josh my diagnosis. He went with me to have the MRI done. He was there when we got home and I listened to the message on the answering machine from my doctor. "*Happy sixteenth birthday, Josh. Your mom has an incurable disease.*"

During the year since then, we've learned a lot about each other. I've learned that my son is responsible, caring, loving, thoughtful, and intelligent. He's stronger than I could ever be, but I gain strength from him. I know that "everything will be okay," because my Josh says it will be, and he cannot be wrong.

We'll count on that, Kathey, for all of us and for all of our children!

10

Beyond "Looking So Good"

There comes a time when MSers have to admit it: we can't look good if we don't feel good. And when we're not comfortable in our clothes, we don't feel good. We might still page through clothing catalogs, weighing the choices for next season's styles, but why bother? After a certain point, the MonSter dictates our fashion imperatives. If we wear anything that's tight, we're going to turn blue from lack of oxygen. If the tightness is at waist level or below, or if belts, buttons, or zippers are involved, we're going to wet our pants before we can make it to the bathroom and undo everything. If we wear shoes that are too high or heavy, we're going to fall on our faces. Just how "good" do we look then?

I used to live in jeans, even wore them to work on days when there were no "dressy" engagements on the calendar. But long before I had any idea that MS had anything to do with it, I realized that my beloved jeans had become instruments of torture. Even when they weren't too tight, they were too stiff and scratchy. They felt more like traps than trappings.

Then the Flutterbuds started talking about clothes. I learned I'm not alone.

Robin Before I had MS, I wore whatever I liked. That is no

longer the case. My skin reactions influence what I wear. My ability to walk affects my choice of clothing and shoes. Weight changes due to the use of steroids and to reduced activity make a big difference. The muscles in my stomach are shot to shit, and that affects how certain articles of clothing fit and feel.

I guess my attitude about what I wear has changed. In terms of relative importance of things in life, the need to be perfectly dressed has lessened. Has anybody else noticed that since having this damned disease?

Kathey   I have. Since this MeSs showed up, I can't stand anything tight or restraining in any way. It's not age- or weight-related; it's just this horrible, constricted feeling, as though I'm being held in and am not... free? I don't know. It's why I haven't worn a belt in years. I can't stand a bra around me either and wouldn't ever wear one if it weren't for the fact that otherwise I'd step on my nipples. I thought for a while it was just because I was getting fatter, but it's not that. Like you, JL, even the loosest tight stuff (like jeans) gets to me. It's like I want to burst out of a shell or get naked!

I'm glad to know this might be an MS thing; well, not really, but you know what I mean. Maybe it's a subconscious reaction, knowing that... well, the clothes are giving us physical clues as to the prison of our bodies? (Okay, that was too deep.)

For me, fashion doesn't matter much. I was never the "high heels" type, anyway. I go with clean, comfortable, and in-good-taste, so I can enjoy what I am doing. To heck with what other people think. Hey, I mean, we look so good anyhow, right?

Bunny   Wow! That's another whole can of worms you opened up there. I never paid attention to this, but guess what? I've been wearing elastic, stretchy-type jeans for more than two years now, because I can't stand being "bound" at the waist. The snap- or button-type jeans went bye-bye a long time ago.

Chris   I love to wear jeans, but most times I find them uncomfortable. The ones that have elastic around the waist fit and feel much better. I also have been buying large shirts, so there's nothing that feels binding!!!!

Vicki   I just found a pair of jeans that fit around my waist without being huge around my butt and legs. I also bought a pair of maternity pants for those days when I'm bloated and nothing fits. The things we do to be comfortable!

Joy   My favorite pants in cool weather are denim leggings. They have just enough spandex to provide some give, and the material is thick enough to hide the less attractive aspects of my legs. They give me the look and feel of jeans, without any binding in the waist or tummy or sagging in the butt. Then I toss on a thigh-length, loose shirt of some kind and pretend I'm thin.

Robin   When I get those pins-and-needles sensations in my legs, leggings seem to act as a buffer between my skin and the world outside. They eliminate the times when a touch, even the sensation of fabric rubbing on my skin, causes a jerk reaction in my legs. Hyper nerves? I'll say!

Helen   I usually wear cotton pants with elastic waists in the summer and sweats in the winter. For the most comfortable things in the world, go to the men's department in one of the discount stores and look for "lounge pants." They're basically pajama bottoms with pockets. They are wonderful!

Sally   I have to get things that are easy to put on. I get exhausted just dressing sometimes. I end up wearing knit pull-on shorts and T-shirts most of the time. When I go out, I wear long pants. There is a place near here that makes lightweight drawstring pants—the kind that tie around the waist and ankles, but otherwise look like hospital scrubs. I replace the ties with elastic, so I can just slip them on without having to fumble with strings. Skirts are hard for me to deal with, because they require a lot of fussing to keep them covering everything and to keep them out of the wheels of my chair. Almost everything I wear is cotton. It's light and absorbent enough to be cool, which is another must for me. Since I live alone, I often wear just my undies on hot days. Once I forgot I just had panties on and opened the door when the UPS guy rang. Oops! Fortunately, it was the nice guy, and we both had a good laugh.

For me, the key words that describe my clothes are: easy, elasticized, no-fuss, cotton, and none.

▲▲▲

This discussion so far gives me an idea. Maybe we should contact the major jeans manufacturers, invite them to contribute heavily to MS research, and point out to them that their sales will increase dramatically when a cure is found.

In the meantime, we'll look at situations where jeans wouldn't be appropriate anyway.

▲▲▲

Bunny I have a dilemma. Paul's company's party is coming up, and I don't have a thing to wear. *Ugh!* What looks kind of fancy but is still comfortable?

Dev When I have to dress up, I wear skirts with elastic tops. I wear shift-type blouses that just cover the tops on the elastic skirts. The combination can look halfway dressy.

Robin I like long dresses with flat boots/shoes. I used to wear a lot of shorter skirts, but these days, I'm so nervous about falling, I'd rather do that in leggings/pants or long dresses.

Me I've made several dressy elastic-waist skirts. Like Robin, I prefer long ones. My all-around favorite apparel, though, are long jumpers with high, gathered waists. They are comfortable, can be dressed up or down depending on what kind of shirt I wear underneath, and are full enough to hide diapers on bad-bladder days. I've even made them for several of the other Flutterbuds.

Kim I still wear your jumpers!

Me No you don't, Kim; you wear the jumpers I made for you.

Kim Oh, yeah, yours wouldn't fit me, would they?

Margo I recently got a pair of "crinkle fabric" pants with an elastic waist. They're very loose and flowing, but not sloppy- or baggy-looking. I wear them with a long pullover sweater. So far, I've worn them to a wedding and a funeral, plus a couple of dinners out.

Ramia Like most other women, I like to look nice whether I'm going out or staying in. I feel bad when I have a day that I spend in pj's and go without a shower. Then that's the last thing my hubby sees before he goes to work and the first thing he sees when he comes home. I want to look nice for him as often as I can.

Vicki Jumpers, pants, tops must pull on, with no buttons.

Ramia I forgot to mention that I curse and carry on at the thought of dealing with buttons.

Me I recently bought a perfectly good denim jumper on sale. I even more recently put it in my Goodwill bag to give it away. "Perfectly good" is no good at all if you can't do the buttons that go all the way down the side (I can't even do enough to get it off and on). And "on sale" is too expensive for something that will just hang in the closet. I'm thinking I should attach a label to it before it goes for resale: "Do not buy this jumper if you have MS."

Helen Everything I own with buttons has been buttoned

once. I just pull shirts, pajamas, or whatever off over my head. The most I have to do or undo is one button each time.

Kim Hey, we are sisters; I do that, too!

Vicki I do, too. Larry laughs because he can tell by the buttons if I wore his shirt last or if he did.

Me Speaking of shirts, I can't wear turtlenecks anymore. I haven't been able to for maybe the past fifteen years. I blame that on fibromyalgia—just the pressure of the cloth sets off pain from my neck down to my hips.

Joy I don't have fibromyalgia, but I can't stand turtlenecks, either, or anything that fits tightly at the neck or waist. I can't even stand elastic on my arms. There's no pain, just a feeling of annoyance and discomfort.

Robin I have this same problem with turtlenecks, unless they're the mock ones that are stretched and don't really touch the skin. You might have a partly-MS thing there, JL, instead of just a fibromyalgia thing.

Margo Me too, but I just thought it was because I'm so much "fluffier" than I used to be. Turtlenecks make me look like... a turtle, I guess. Plus the tightness issue and the "I'm too hot" issue....

Nadiza Now this goes to show you just how important we are to each other. I had no idea that others had this same problem. It's not like it's in any books about MS. Of course, after this it will be! If it weren't for us discussing this, many other MSers would think they were nuts or imagining it.

Robin How about shoes? I have to wear flat shoes and finding nice flats is a real challenge. I found a couple pairs in basic colors that will go with all my pants. But dressy flats? I haven't found those. There's a real lack of good stuff for people who don't want to wear the "college fashions," especially in shoes.

Me Do you know where I usually buy shoes? I hate to admit it, but K-Mart has cheap ones that are so unfashionable, there's no way they qualify as the college kind. They're flat, unadorned, and just what I need!

Kathey You betcha! And those little WalMart flat, tie-up, canvas tennies are the best! (I have pink and yellow and turquoise and purple and black and white and, well, you get the drift.) Also the best—my "shoestrings." I bought these things that look like twisty phone cords. You lace them into the shoes and never have to tie them or worry about them coming untied or being too loose or too tight. They turn your tie shoes into slip-ons.

Sharon That's a ditto. I live in my sneakers, and they have those stretchy laces. But I can tie now since the surgery, so I'm going to get me some grown-up shoes!

Sally I can't feel the floor through shoes to know if my foot is down right or if I'm about to twist my ankle again. So I am barefoot unless I have to wear *something* on my feet, and then it is knit booties just for looks. I saw a pair of thin moccasins that might work. They have no soles other than the same thin leather the tops are made of, so I should be able to feel the floor when I wear them (fingers crossed).

Vicki I usually wear tennis shoes. If I have to go somewhere dressy, I wear those elastic, silky house slippers. I've also been known to just wear socks to the stores. I'm always in my wheelchair, so it really doesn't matter what is on my feet.

Joy I look for shoes that are not just flat, but also heavily cushioned, as with a quarter-inch rubber sole. My feet and legs tire and ache so much, so I like to put something between them and the hard floors.

Okay, we've figured out what to wear. Now what do we do about the rest of our appearance? How about taking care of hair (on our heads and elsewhere), makeup, and the even more personal "have to" concerns?

My hair has always been my biggest gripe. It's superfine and superstraight. I used to think that keeping it short would make it easier to care for. But it grows in seventy-seven opposing directions, so I ended up looking much too tousled all the time. Now it's longer, so its own weight keeps it anchored in the direction in which I set it. I usually wash it in the shower at night; then in the morning I dampen it slightly and do a once-over with a blow dryer and curling iron. That's fast and easy enough to forestall arm fatigue.

Tara   That's like me. I have finally decided to just keep my hair straight. I usually wash it and let it dry almost all the way before I get the blow dryer and finish it. I dry it with my head upside-down; hold onto the countertop or you may end up looking up at it. When an MSer goes upside down, the rest of the person's body takes a while to adapt to that position. Usually the body insists on resting on the floor while this is taking place.

Chris   I have started to just not do a thing with mine. It looks fine to me, and I don't have the energy to do things like I used to!!! I wash my hair in the shower, too. That's easier than bending over a sink!!!

Bunny   That's a sore subject! I used to stand in front of the mirror with my handy-dandy curling iron and can of hairspray for an hour. I don't have the stamina for that anymore. Now I try to keep it permed and just wash and go. It seems to be the easiest for me. Especially since Paul wants me to keep it long, and I look yucky with straight hair.

149

Ramia How can you put your hair in a simple ponytail at those times when you are home but your left arm is whooping it up in Acapulco? When ponytails got too tough to do, I got a haircut. All I do is step out of the shower, towel dry, then comb with my fingers. I'd like to let it grow out again, though, if I could figure out how to take care of it.

Sharon I gave up on ponytails a long time ago and had my hair cut shorter. I used to love to do it up in buns and tails and put in combs. But when my tremor got bad, trying to use my left arm to do my hair only resulted in me slapping myself in the head. I've got Joy to do that for me now!

Robin Instead of ponytails, use those banana clips that can pull your hair back in just an easy clip. With a little practice, they work great. They're also good for keeping your neck cool in the summer!

Debby Those headbands with the zigzag teeth are wonderful. I can put one in, and it holds up my hair and bangs and looks stylish. I've found a hairdresser who gives me a good cut each time and helps me with styles that don't involve a lot of work or that don't require my arms to be up for a long time. He knows about the MS, too, and is careful about the products he uses on me and takes notes on my reactions to different products. That helps.

Joy Another thing worth mentioning: the newer shampoo chairs in beauty shops are horrible! They are not comfortable, and I'm always afraid that when my head goes back into that position, I will have an attack of vertigo. So I shampoo at home before I get a cut. I color my hair at home, too. To rinse, I kneel on the floor, lean forward over the tub, and use a hand-held shower attachment. That way I am already close to the floor, so if I get dizzy, I don't have far to fall!

Helen I have wash-and-wear hair. I've always worn my hair short but have found since MS that extremely short works the best. I cut the top with a one-inch spacer on the clippers, the sides and back with a half-inch one.

The makeup manufacturers might want to join in the search for a cure for MS, too. I used to wear it almost all the time—it just made me feel better about myself. Now it's reserved for special occasions. I do okay with the basics—foundation and blush and gloss—that don't require rock-steady hands. For the mascara, my hands usually just rock, and I end up poking myself in the eye with the wand. I have to engage in a lot of arm-propping to get it right.

Bunny This is another sore subject with me. I used to wear makeup all the time. Now I don't wear it at all, unless I'm getting dressed up to go to a party or something to that effect. When I do use it, I stick with simple.

Kathey I started using pancake makeup about six months ago. You apply it with a damp makeup sponge. It has eliminated the problems I had with foundation, since my right hand isn't very coordinated, and I have so little feeling in my fingertips. Mascara is a must for me; I think I look tiny-eyed without it. I've been lucky so far to not have many problems with mascara, but I keep a damp cotton swab handy for "boo-boos."

Helen When I have to use makeup, it's a bit of foundation, a bit of blush, some eye shadow and some mascara, period. So far, so good. I can still put a new paint job on the old chassis!

Debby It is just too cruel for me to go out in public without makeup on. The world doesn't deserve that. I was having a hard time with foundations, because my hands didn't work well enough to blend it. I finally found a powdered mineral foundation. It goes on sheer, with great coverage, and I just use a big old brush to put it on. I rest my arm on the dresser while doing the mascara. My whole makeup routine takes only about three minutes. I make sure I do that every day, because then I just feel better overall.

Laura I had a terrible time brushing my teeth. So I bought a battery-operated toothbrush. I started with a kid's one; now I have a bigger one, but I still travel with the small one.

Debby I use an electric toothbrush, too; that is much easier than trying to hold onto a regular one. I use floss called Glide®, because it doesn't get stuck in my teeth and makes it go much quicker.

Me I have trouble flossing when my hands are numb. I can't hold onto the floss and can't manipulate it through the areas it has to go through. Joe, my dentist, recommended that I use those wooden interdental stimulators. They're like fat, flat toothpicks, easier to hold onto than floss. He also said that, for any of his patients who have conditions or are on medications that could affect their dental health, he recommends taking advantage of all the gadgets that have popped up on the market recently for oral hygiene: electric toothbrushes, sonar toothbrushes, the little water sprayers, and the like. Well, ladies, we all know what bladder-control medications (not to mention a whole pharmacopeia of other stuff that we take) do to our mouths. Dry! I think I'll add one or two of his recommendations to my next Christmas list.

Robin You know how the heat from a warm shower makes us tired and weak? I hate cold showers! So I do my warm shower, then I get out and put a towel on the toilet (we have a really small bathroom, so the toilet is right next to the tub) and sit down to dry. I keep things like deodorant, moisturizer, and comb within easy reach. Then I take a ten-minute break while doing my personal things.

Janis I have to lean or at least touch the wall when I shower. As soon as I shut my eyes, my body forgets where it is. And when I turn around, I have to go slowly. It's like my head turns one way, but my eyes and the rest of my body face in the direction they started out for a few seconds longer. Weird! As for me shaving my legs, well, let's just say that weebles wobble and they do fall down! I am thinking of getting an electric shaver for my legs. But I still have to use a razor because I shave "other" areas, too.

Chris I shave my legs while sitting on the toilet and putting my legs on the edge of the tub.

Debby When I shave my legs, I usually stand in the shower with my leg propped up on the back of the tub. I have a hard time getting a good grip on the razor, so I have cut a wash-cloth into strips; I wrap a strip around the handle to give me more control and cut down on cuts.

Kathey Shaving legs? Oh that's so much fun (not!). I can manage, usually, by leaning back against the wall of the shower and putting one foot at a time up on the opposite tub rim. Electric shavers would eliminate a lot of cuts, I'm sure. And, there are always the chemical hair removers. They do work [if you're not sensitive to the ingredients—I am!], and it's easy to just slather them on, wait the allotted time, then rinse.

Kim No matter what I try or how I try, I just can't get this one right. I can manage to shave the fronts of my legs, but I can't reach around with a good enough aim to shave the backs.

Me Tink, have you tried standing behind yourself? Then you just have to reach down in front of you.

Kim Now why didn't I think of that? I guess I was beside myself. Another thing that's nearly impossible is cutting toenails. I am almost to the point of having my friend Rita do them for me. Gads, it's hell getting old. Or feeble. Or both.

Chris Gee, I thought I was the only one having trouble doing that!

Me Far from it, Chris. I have trouble with that, too. My clippers go wherever they want to when I try to get them into the right places. I end up either cutting air or clipping into my toe. Meanwhile, I'm trying to keep my foot steady, while it's sitting there spazzing out, propped up on the opposite knee, which isn't too steady either. Maybe I should try sitting on the floor to clip my toenails. As far as I know, the floor is steady.

Helen I've learned that cutting my toenails in the tub is possible if I open the drain a little so that the clippings go down, and I'm not sitting on them. The same goes for shaving my legs and armpits.

Donna I keep a barstool, without arms or back, in the bathroom. I use it to get me through all my personal care. I lean over it when I dry my hair and let it support my weight. The stool is the right height for me to sit on while I brush my teeth, fix my hair and apply makeup. I can see myself in the bathroom mirror and the makeup mirror I keep on the windowsill, and I can reach the necessary drawers or shelves easily.

Dev I try to take care of myself the simplest and best way I can. But I am a stickler on always being clean and well groomed, even when I'm running around the house in an old pair of sweatpants and a flannel shirt. I even put on my favorite cologne every day. Somehow, it always makes me feel better. I smell good, besides looking good!

Me   I do the same thing, Dev. I have maybe a half-dozen bottles of those lightly scented body sprays and use them according to what mood I'm in. That way I never get tired of smelling myself.

Which reminds me of a new topic. Some time ago, I read that the ultimate humiliation is discovering that you're no longer able to wipe your own ass. I jokingly mentioned it to the Flutterbuds. But I found out that it's no joke.

Bunny   Wiping has become a big problem for me. Any suggestions? I know this is a gross subject, but it's a real problem.

Vicki   I'd suggest you use lots of toilet paper. You know, the bigger the bundle, the shorter the distance to your target. If you're still having trouble: baby wipes, baby wipes, baby wipes. Put them in a plastic bag when you finish using them; then throw them away.

Me   Those soft cotton pads that come soaked in witch hazel, you know, the ones that are supposed to relieve hemorrhoid irritation? Those work well for cleansing delicate areas, too. But again, I don't know if they can be flushed. (I used them right after having each of my babies. But I don't have any around now to check the labels.)

Robin   I seem to remember that some manufacturer now makes wet wipes that are flushable? [Just be sure they aren't the antibacterial kind. Ouch!] I can't say I've ever tried them, but they're supposed to work well on babies.

Kim   Yes! I got a case of them for about eleven dollars. They are so soft and smell like baby lotion. At least, once I get cleaned up, my ass smells good!

Could Kim be trying to come up with the perfect response for the next time somebody says, "But you look so good!"?— "No, I don't. But once I get cleaned up..."!

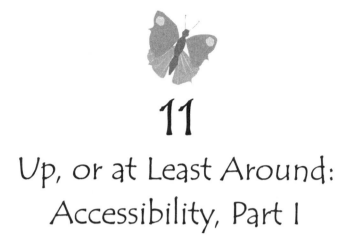

11

Up, or at Least Around: Accessibility, Part I

In *Women Living with Multiple Sclerosis*, the ladies in our Froup talked about the need for using assistive devices to enable us to remain ambulatory or at least mobile. At that time, many of us were new to the concept of needing any kind of assistance, and our concern was mostly for the emotional issues involved. We hated the idea that hanging onto canes or crutches or sitting in wheelchairs would label us as "handicapped." We worried about the impact these aids would have on our families, friends, co-workers, and others close to us. This time we touch on those issues, but only briefly. The original Flutterbuds have had a couple of years to adjust to the whole idea. The new ladies in the group, some of whom have more recently reached a point where they need help with getting around, are eager to exchange views on the subject and to learn which devices have been most helpful for us. They're interested in choosing and using these devices wisely and effectively.

Debby I guess I should tell all of you; I broke down and bought a cane today. I haven't used it yet, but buying it is at least a step forward to acceptance, if not yet a literal step forward on my feet.

Joy   That's like me and my cheap, folding wheelchair in the garage. I bought it "just in case." I've rarely used it. We're just being prepared, like the Boy Scouts, right?

Debby   It felt a little odd to go in and buy the cane, but I ran into an old friend and she asked me if I had started celebrating New Year's early, because I was a little off balance. It made me so mad, I went right out and bought it before I had a chance to think more about it. I will not be accused of being a lush. So, I have the cane, and it sits in my bedroom. It's not completely useless, though. It makes a dang nice hook to catch the kids with!

Dev   Good for you, Debby. Yes, that is a big step forward. Now use it when you need it. Don't be stubborn like me. I could have prevented a lot of falls if I had just used my cane.

Robin   I hear you! When I bought mine, it sat in the car for a few weeks before I got up the courage to use it. It felt really weird to use in the beginning. Now I like it. It's an adjustable one, with dense foam on the handle—very comfy to hold!
   Don't worry, Debby. When you're ready, you'll use yours.

Dev   I used mine all evening on Christmas Eve. It was actually the first time I'd ever let my girls see me use it. When I was sitting, I would prop it in the corner next to me. The only thing one of them said was, "Look, Santa Claus was here!" Everyone laughed, and that was it.

Robin   That's what's kind of silly about the whole thing. It's much less of an issue to others than we think it is. If it's an issue to us, it's for a whole host of different reasons, independence being one of them. It's not really the cane that bothers us, but the implications behind it.

Kathey A couple of months ago, Josh and I were at the drugstore waiting for a prescription to be filled. While we waited, we looked at the "assistive devices," because we'd been thinking that my mom should get a shower chair. Then Josh pointed to the canes and said, "I bet you could walk farther and straighter with one of these." We looked them over, found the one I liked best, and we bought it. Josh didn't realize the emotional impact it had on me to get it. But because he'd been the one to suggest it, I was able to temper my "Holy shit, why do I need that?" feelings.

I haven't used it much so far, except around the house. Josh just takes it all in stride (no pun intended). This will help me do more of what I love to do (walk). So buying it was the right decision.

Now I just have to latch onto some of Josh's attitude. My using a cane is not a big issue for him.

Robin You know, I've found out that it's no big deal when people see me with my cane and ask why I'm using it. It doesn't even embarrass me anymore. I simply say, "I have MS," and either the subject is dropped right there, or the person I'm talking with asks questions about it. I've ended up having some interesting conversations as a result. My cane is turning out to be an icebreaker for lots of people.

Me Isn't it nice to be able to be helpful? You see somebody about to walk on a patch of ice, you say, "Hey, wait a minute!" Then you rush over and break the ice with your cane and everybody can walk safely! Good work, Robin!

Robin Gee, thanks, JL! Leave it to you to find more than one use for the things we need! Did you know the cane is also useful for smacking smart-asses?

Joy I'm not sure a cane would help me much. When I'm off balance or a bit dizzy, I prefer to have something more substantial—and less likely to be moved by me—to hang onto. Like Jack's arm, a stair-rail, a shopping cart, a wall, furniture, even the corner of a mantle, just to provide a sort of grip on reality and steady me, not to bear my weight.

Vicki When I'm dizzy or way off balance, the cane doesn't help much. I also prefer using walls or chairs for balance. If I use the cane when I'm like that, I find myself walking in circles around the cane.

Joy Do y'all know how to use a cane properly? What is the right height for a cane? I ask because I know some of the Buds have discussed this before, and it apparently isn't as simple as it seems it would be. Maybe somebody could jump in here with some pointers learned from physical therapists?

Dev Joy, at first, I had a bad time with the cane. It kept getting in my way; I was actually tripping over it. The first one I got was too short. It made me stoop over while I walked, and my shoulder was killing me. The one I have now is waist-high and seems to work better for me. I tried them both out, just walking around the house, and I definitely do better with the taller one. It actually helps me stand straighter.

Kim While working in a physical therapy clinic as a kid, I learned that you're supposed to use the cane on the opposite side of the one you are having problems with.

Robin That's interesting. My right leg is the weaker—but sometimes it's easier to use the cane on that side. When I'm standing on my left leg, picking up my right foot is hard, especially when I'm tired. I feel the tiredness more in that leg. It's okay to stand on either leg with the cane in either hand. But when I'm walking, it helps my balance to have the extra point of support on the right while I'm picking up and moving my right leg. Did that make any sense at all? Sheesh! Whoever said this would be simple?

Dev I do the opposite, Robin. I'm left-handed, so it's hard for me to control the cane with my right hand. I lead with my right leg but hold the cane with my left hand. When I first started using it, I would hold the cane in my left hand and try to lead with my left leg because it is my stronger side. But that's why I kept tripping over it. It really was something new to learn.

Margo When I got mine, the salesman fitted it to rest comfortably in my hand, so that I don't have to either bend my elbow or hold my arm straight down. I walk with it in my right hand, in sync with my right leg. And, yes, I often have to stop and restart my stride to be sure the cane moves with my right foot. However, using the cane does cause fatigue in the arm/wrist/shoulder, so you want to be careful of that and make sure the one you get is adjusted properly.

The point is, you can really wear yourself out if you don't know how to use it. If somebody isn't available to teach you, my suggestion would be to first practice around the house. I got one of those canes that is shaped like a seven, with an almost 90-degree handle on it. It's adjustable, which is nice, but it's kind of uncomfortable on my hand. It does make a nice door unlocker; when Roy lets me into the truck first, I can use it to reach over and unlock his door for him.

Kathey I don't know if yours is like mine, Margo, but from your description, I guess it is. Not a "hook," but with a flat top? Here's a hint: Don't hold it with the point facing backwards; hold it with the point facing forwards, so that your shoulder takes the brunt of the force, not your wrist and arm.

Kim I can only use round-handled canes. The ones that look like a seven really added a lot of stress to my arm and wrist. When I went to the old-fashioned rounded cane, the pain stopped immediately.

161

Kathey I think the most important thing is to get a cane that supports you enough. Then hold it in whatever way feels right to you (assuming that's possible; it still feels awkward to me, emotionally more than physically, to use it at all). I would worry more about the right height and size than about what hand to hold it in. You want to feel confident that, if you stumble, the cane will support you. The last thing any of us needs is to have the cane cause a screwed-up shoulder or wrist or elbow on our "good" side!

Dev I have trouble carrying things and holding onto a cane at the same time. I'm in the habit of just hanging the cane on my arm when I have to carry something, so I have both hands free. But then I have to walk very slowly because I have an armful of stuff and no support. I haven't learned how to carry things and use it at the same time. Any suggestions?

Me After all these years, I still haven't learned the trick, Dev. When I go out of the house at all (if I'm walking instead of sitting in the wheelchair), I use both crutches, so I can't carry anything. I wear a waist pack instead of carrying a purse, which helps some. Anything that doesn't fit in there just can't go with me. I've tried carrying things in a tote hooked over my shoulder or on my arm. But it's hard to move the crutches with something hanging down and bumping into them. I think I'm going to invent something like those baby carriers that can be worn front or back, but stiffer, so that whatever you have to carry doesn't spill or get squished. Maybe a kind of basket that hooks around the waist?

Margo Why isn't there a "fanny pack" that doesn't look completely dorky? That would help me out a lot, but they look so dumb, especially on a fanny that has plenty of packing on it already. (No offense to anyone. I just don't care for the way they look....)

Kim   I use a fanny pack, dorky or not.

Vicki   I use a backpack. There's more room in those than in a fanny pack.

Me   So now we have a fanny pack, a backpack, and a waist pack. Does anybody want to try a nose pack? How about hanging our purses from our ears? I tried carrying a purse with my teeth but couldn't concentrate on walking and clenching my jaws at the same time. What are we to do?

Margo   Here's another question: how do you dig your checkbook, etc., out of a backpack without a world of trouble? The only thing I've come up with that works for me (and it doesn't work very well, or I wouldn't be having all these problems) is to carry my checkbook and pen in my back jeans' pocket and my keys in my front jeans' pocket, hang my sunglasses off the front of my T-shirt, carry my smokes in my shirt pocket (well, I guess I could roll them up in my sleeve), and put anything else in my other jeans' pockets. That works when I can remember to grab everything I need when I leave the house, remember which pocket everything is in, remember to put it all away when I get home again, and remember to never, ever wear sweatpants. I get so confused!

Me   My waist pack has lots of little compartments. I'm very strict about where things end up in there, so that when I need something, I know just where to go for it. Space is at a minimum, so I know I'd better use it wisely and carry only what I'll absolutely need. That works well for me, because I used to be a purse packrat. When I went out, I'd stuff things I thought I might need into my purse; while I was out, I'd toss in more stuff that I wanted to take home. Then I'd promptly forget they were in there, until the purse got too fat to carry. Talk about fatigue in the arms and shoulders! The waist pack doesn't cause any muscle strain, and, since I carry it on the front, I can get to the contents easily.

Vicki If I have to write a check, I dig. The backpack rides on the arms of my wheelchair; I just reach around and grab it. When I could walk better, I would do what Margo does. I'd carry the checkbook only—most stores have a pen to use. Then I'd either hook the cane on my arm or lean it against the counter while I wrote.

Dee I am at a loss about trying to use my cane. I cannot use it anymore; it's just too hard on my arms and shoulders. I can use a wheelchair if there's someone to push it, but the only kind I could use on my own would have to be motorized. I don't think a walker would work, either, because I don't have the strength to lift it up and move it along.

Margo Dee, I am so there! It seems that I'm getting weaker every damned day! My cane is almost becoming a hazard. I lose my balance even when I use it, and I find myself kicking it all the time. I'm not sure I could successfully navigate a walker. I mean, if I'm tripping over a cane, can you imagine me with a walker? I hate to even try the forearm crutches, but I guess that's the next step.

Me Dee and Margo, this is exactly why I got my forearm crutches. A couple of years ago, I lost a lot of strength all at once: in my arms, legs, torso, all over my body. I couldn't walk more than a few steps even with my canes. They didn't give me enough support, and I had trouble picking them up and moving them. I was sure that I'd be in a wheelchair all the time before long. Then I decided to try the crutches. When I first started using them, I guess I handled them like canes; I let most of my weight fall on the hand rests. That made me hyperextend my wrists, and it hurt! So I made padded covers for the handles and reminded myself to rely more on the arm attachments than the hand rests to support me. That did the trick! It was as if somebody had handed me a miracle! I could walk again, more than just a few steps, with no pain or instant fatigue.

Kim I couldn't agree more! Mine are my best buddies; I couldn't get along without them.

Dee I think that's the way I am going to go. If I start using my cane again, the pain I'd been having in my shoulders will start up again. It does help to get the doctor to write a prescription, doesn't it? I mean to get insurance coverage for them.

Me It depends on your insurance, Dee. Mine requires a $100 co-payment for durable medical equipment; then it pays a percentage of the cost over that. Guess what? The crutches cost $100! So the insurance didn't pay anything on them. But we got them through a local health supplies place that offers a 15 percent discount to MSers. We ended up getting them for $85. They're worth every cent of it, too!

Dee I guess what I keep doubting about the forearm crutches is that I'll have the strength to use them.

Me That's the great thing about them. The weaker you are, the better they work. The harder you lean into them, the more they support you. It's almost as if there's a person on either side of you, holding you up by your arms.

Robin Don't they do a number on your arms and shoulders, though? I imagine that would tire them out a lot.

Me Isn't there a law of physics that says that for every action, there's an equal and opposite reaction? If there isn't, there should be, because that seems to be the way the crutches work. You can just let your weight rest on the crutches—there's no effort involved on your part. The crutches "react" by pushing up on your arms, giving you whatever measure of support your weight indicates you need. Then, since the crutches are hooked securely onto your forearms, you just have to guide them by the handles, and they stay with you wherever you go. Again, there's no effort on your part, no need to grip them with your hands and lift them every time you take a step. They've been my best means of avoiding fatigue when I want to walk instead of ride.

Robin How about using a scooter for times when you can't walk? One catalog I saw even has a scooter equipped with carriers for crutches that you could use when you want to get up and walk. I think they're about half the price of power wheelchairs.

Me For most of us, that would probably depend again on how much of the cost our insurance would cover. I've heard some weird stories about that from other MSers. For example, one lady on the message boards asked her insurance company for a little scooter. They denied her request but instead bought her a huge power wheelchair (which cost at least twice as much as a scooter, Robin!). She doesn't have room to use it in her house, and it doesn't fold, so it can't be put into her car trunk. It's basically useless, as far as she's concerned. I guess the best thing to do is to figure out what kind of equipment will be helpful to you, considering the accessibility of your house and what means of transporting it you'll have. Ask your doctor to document that the specific device would be most helpful for you. Then request that the insurance company pay for something that meets those recommendations while falling within its criteria for coverage.

Kathey I think so often about asking the doctor for a prescription for a scooter. I don't know what's holding me back, except...okay, gang, this is stupid, but I keep thinking that folks will think, "Look at that chubby girl; she's too lazy to walk." I suppose that even if I lost fifty pounds, I would find some other excuse. Using a scooter is such a big change.

But the moment the MonSter robs me of my walks (especially in the zoo!), I'll be motorized!

Me   Kathey, if anybody thinks anything at all about you being in a scooter (and being "chubby," if that's the way you want to put it), they'll probably just think that you haven't been able to exercise because you aren't able to walk. Besides, who cares what anybody thinks? You know you're not lazy, we know you're not lazy, and that's all that counts, right?

Dev   Ah, Kathey, your attitude is contagious! The kids are talking about going to the Home and Flower Show, and they want me to go, too. I told them that it would be too difficult, because my legs would get too tired. Stef said, "Mom, they have scooters there; just get one!" I asked her if she would be embarrassed and she said, "Heck, no! Besides, you'd be able to see more without having to worry about getting tired." I've never used a scooter, but the stiffness and spasms in my legs when I have to do a lot of walking are telling me it's time. There have been so many times my family wanted me to do something that required a lot of walking, and I refused, all because of my stupid pride. I've decided it's time to let that go! So we are starting out with the scooter at the Home & Flower Show, and if I don't run over anybody, we'll plan other outings!

Dee   I know it is really hard to think of things like actually buying a scooter. However, I try to think that having those assistive devices would help me to be able to participate in things that I wouldn't get to if I didn't use them.

Helen   Once you get past the point of cussing because you need one, scooters are fun. I love mine! They move faster than the average person walks; so you have to actually slow down to keep pace with whomever you are with, which can be kind of empowering, right? And no matter where you are, when you're on a scooter, you never have to look for a seat.

167

Also, for those of you who like to explore woods or beaches or hilly places, some scooters will handle rough terrain quite well. Check with manufacturers or dealers to see which have tires suitable for different surfaces.

I've never tried to buy a scooter or a power chair. I was lucky that a friend of my mom had a scooter that she no longer needed, so she passed it on to me. It has an extra battery on it, which makes it too heavy for Ron to lift into our van (that's where a ramp or lift on the van would come in handy). But we live a couple of blocks from a shopping center, and I can use the scooter to go there by myself. I get such a feeling of freedom every time I do that!

My insurance company did buy me a new manual wheelchair (after I paid the first $100, plus a percentage of the balance). It's tiny (I don't want to have to move around a ton of extra metal to get it to move me around!), lightweight, and rolls almost effort-lessly, even when there's nobody to push me. That's rare, though—Ron thinks it's neat to have an excuse to push me around! Even my girls can lift it easily in or out of their cars when I go some-place with them.

A final thought on the subject: If your insurance company won't help to purchase assistive devices (canes, crutches, walkers, wheelchairs, scooters), check with your local chapter of the National Multiple Sclerosis Society. Many of them have special funds set up or donations earmarked to provide this kind of help. Sometimes the NMSS will cooperate with Medicare or insurance companies to cover the full cost.

Tara   I got my power wheelchair through vocational rehab when I was still working. It cost $17,000!

Dee   That had to be for more than a wheelchair, didn't it?

Please tell me it was for more than one wheelchair.

Tara It was just for the chair. But my chair has a tilt mechanism, so I don't have to wear myself out just trying to sit up. It also has two batteries, the best cushion system there is, and so on. It was custom made to fit me, because I'm so tall. So the price reflects all those add-ons.

Sometimes all the canes and wheelchairs in the world won't do us much good, even as we try to get around our own houses. That's when we have to look for other ways just to move our bodies to where we want to go.

Dev I can't go down stairs at all anymore, unless I have a railing or someone to hang onto. My balance has gotten much worse in the past year.

Joy Fortunately, the only stairs I must deal with now are the ones to our attic, which I don't have to use very often and which have a railing for me to hang onto. I simply don't attempt any stairs, anywhere, unless they have handrails. Even then, I take it slowly and carefully and go either barefoot or in tennis shoes, so I can feel the steps. I've been known to have the ol' foot drop problem, too, which doesn't make it easy to do steps. Heck, I recently stumbled over the marble inlay in front of our fireplace—it's all of a quarter-inch high!—and came close to falling on my face. Just call me clumsy, but careful.

Vicki I know the feeling all too well. When you do fall, of course, it's always in areas where there's no furniture or anything to grab onto to hoist yourself up. Which means you have to do the G.I. Joe crawl to get somewhere to be able to get up.

Helen Thanks to my military training, I can do this quite well. If I get down on the floor to attach yet another part to the computer, I have to scoot over to the desk to haul my fat ass up again. I swear, I just should get a skateboard and stay down on the floor. The worst for me, though, is going up the stairs. I go up on all fours. What's that book about "everything I needed to know, I learned from my dog"? That's me!

Dee I've had to do this for the last two weeks at our son's house. It is a split-level and our room is downstairs. On all fours is the only way to make it upstairs; I sit on my bottom to get down sometimes.

Helen Dee, I do that every morning! I could probably make it on my feet, but I have to carry two of the pups down to let them out. It goes something like this: Okay, Chance in my right hand, T'Belle in my left hand; that works, yes. But, wait a minute here—how in hell am I going to hang onto the rail? So, down on my butt I go, with two doglets in my arms, and I bump, bump, bump down the stairs. Now, you'd think this would firm up the big butt, wouldn't you? Not!

Kathey Bumpin' down the stairs.... We used to do that for fun when I was a kid. I bet it's not fun anymore, though.

Me I have a harder time balancing when I'm going down steps than when I'm going up. It's as if I get top-heavy all of a sudden. I just can't keep my body aligned the right way.

Joy I've heard others say that, too. But I don't think that's my problem. With me, it is weakness in the legs more than lack of balance. (Although I've been known to butt-crawl down the stairs on dizzy days, too!)

Bunny I'm going to tell you all about what I've been using to help with balance. Magnets! I started wearing magnetic insoles in my shoes and slippers, and they are definitely helping my balance.

Robin Tell me more, Bunny. Balance is one of my biggest problems.

Bunny Okay, Robin. You asked for it! Basically, these magnets are designed to work with your own body's chemistry to promote balance and well-being. When I first tried them, I did the usual "close your eyes and fall over" test for the guy who came to demonstrate them. You should have seen this guy's face when I immediately tipped over! Then I put the insoles on and closed my eyes. Did I fall? Nope! I still wavered, but not as badly. These are not a cure-all, but they do promote stability.

Paul and I are so happy with the way they've helped me that we have become distributors of these products. He has known about them for quite some time and has wanted insoles for himself for work. He works on concrete floors all day long, and the docs were talking about knee surgery for him. Now that he's wearing the insoles, he's no longer in pain. I wear the socks and the insoles and am doing much better. At least it's something to help me get through my daily activities.

Chris I lose my balance so often, my cane doesn't help at all, and I really don't think that magnets or anything else would help, either. I don't want to have to start using crutches or a wheelchair. It's hopeless!

Jamie It is not, Chris! There are more options than just a cane. You might have to push your pride out of the way for a little while. But when you find the best thing to help you get around without falling, then your pride will come back. It will mean that you took control from the MonSter and that you're going to live as comfortably and safely as you can.

Kim I've been thinking about getting a wheelchair. I know the day is getting closer when I'll really need one. I don't deal with changes very well and using a wheelchair would be a big change. But at least I'm not alone!

Jamie I went from being paralyzed to using a wheelchair, to a cane, to forearm crutches, to a walker, back to forearms again, and now I'm up to the walker on wheels that has a little seat (I can flip it down and sit when I get too weak to walk). I use a wheelchair for big trips like grocery shopping. I've been through just about everything there is, so I (and most of the other ladies here) all know the pain and depression that comes with any change in strength. We all do what we have to do to adapt, even if it doesn't appeal to us. Just remember you are still "you" on the inside. It's okay to mourn a loss, and we've all lost a lot no matter what stage we are in. But our Higher Power gives us the strength, the drive, and the desire to live as independently as we can. And he gave us each other so that we are never alone in this fight against the MonSter.

Well said, Jamie. We'll keep your words in mind when even bigger changes, meaning more adaptations, come along.

Chris I've changed so much that I can't even take a shower by myself now. I've fallen trying to get out of the shower, not once, but twice, in the past couple of days. Mike has to help me out every time. You should see my bruises!

Kim Did I tell you gals that I got a shower chair? That's something for you to consider, Chris.

Vicki Aren't they great? I just got a new one. My first one must have had a weight limit on it, and I must have gone over the limit, because the legs started spreading. My new one has a back to it, which holds it together better.

Chris I don't have trouble while I'm taking my shower. I shower in the tub, and I fall when I try to get out. Mike and I were talking about what we can do to make it easier. We thought maybe one of those rails on the side of the tub would help. I'm going to try that; it can't hurt!

Kathey Absolutely! They're great even for people who don't have problems with strength or balance. And please, think again about getting a shower chair. It's not the prettiest thing in the world, but neither is your bruised body, Chris! (I meant the bruises aren't pretty—I'm sure your body is beautiful!). If you get a shower chair, you can sit down and dry off before you get out of the tub.

The simple things are so important. How about using a nonslip bathmat? Install handrails wherever they might come in handy. Every little safety feature that you can come up with will help.

Chris Okay! I've heard enough now! I will be more careful and I will sit down while drying off! And I will get used to the changes.

Margo We remodeled the bathroom about four years ago. That was back in my "what's wrong with me?" stage. I asked Roy to put in grab bars at the time, but in his own sense of denial, I guess, he just blew that request off. Now, if we put them in, we'll have to drill through my English tile, and frankly, it pisses me off.

Me Margo, you might not have to destroy your English tile. I've seen freestanding grab bars/support rails in catalogs. They're built in the shape of a U, so they're designed to fit around your commode. But there's no law that says you can't use them wherever they'd be most helpful.

We redid our bathroom last year as part of our general attempt to make our house wheelchair accessible. It was tiny, with hardly enough room to stand in there, much less to maneuver a wheelchair in and out. So we enlarged it by a foot in the width. We took out the tub and replaced it with a shower stall that's very easy to get in and out of. I use a chair every time I shower. I think I could easily transfer directly from my wheelchair to my shower chair if I ever have to. Ron installed grab bars, both in the shower and on the wall outside of it. It's great now! Taking a shower used to be a scary experience, but I feel much more secure with the new design.

Laura This talk about making our houses accessible reminds me of when we bought our condo (really a townhome). There were three styles available: two different two-story ones and a ranch. I really liked one of the two-story ones; Hubby liked the ranch. He pointed out to me that I sometimes had trouble with stairs at our old house, and if things should get worse, a ranch would be better. That's dirty pool, using my MS to get his way, isn't it?

Kim It most certainly is dirty pool! Gads, I just hate it when someone else is right.

The rest of the remodeling that Ron and I did last year included enlarging all the inside doorways to thirty-six inches wide, which allows enough space to turn a wheelchair slightly to aim for the hall while going through the doorway. That avoids smashing into the opposite wall on the way. The biggest change was putting a ten-foot addition onto our bedroom (there was hardly room to get our bodies to the bed before; there would have been no way to get around it in a wheelchair). We installed double sliding glass doors on the back wall of the bedroom, with a wheelchair ramp just outside of them.

I hated to go through the expense and hassle of doing a complete makeover to our house, but once I accepted the idea that we had to do it, I discovered some nice surprises. I used to feel kind of claustrophobic in this house, because the rooms were all so boxy, with little bitty doorways in between. Now we have more than enough space to be comfortable, and we can sit in one room without feeling completely closed off from the rest of the house.

Last but not least, when we made our plans for the remodeling, I typed a list of everything we felt we should do. I took the list to Dr. Reed, and he signed it, indicating that he recommended all the changes we'd outlined. That meant that, when it came time to file our income tax return for the year, we were able to claim all the authorized expenses as medical deductions (within the IRS's limitations, of course). That was a nice bonus and helped to offset some of the cost of the work.

It was one more time that the MonSter made me do something I didn't want to do, and then I ended up being able to thumb my nose at It! Thanks again, MonSter!

Margo I've given tons of thought to "universally accessible" designs. I've designed a house with many features that I think are simply good planning for anyone in this day and age. All the doors are four feet wide. There is broad use of pocket doors, so there's no problem with swinging them open or closed. All the spaces are large, without feeling cavernous. Yes, it has stairs, also four feet wide. My thought is that any new home could be designed with stairs as long as the lift mechanism is built in from the beginning, instead of being retrofitted at a later date. The light switches, of course, are the rocker-type and located low enough to be reached from a wheelchair; electrical outlets are located high enough for the same usage. My house (and you know, of course, that it's a log house) also has an elevator running from the basement to

175

the loft. That's not just a matter of accessibility. I mean, who wants to move a queen-sized bed up a set of stairs?

"My" kitchen has a fridge with the freezer on the bottom and a generous lowered work area, equipped for a person in a wheelchair to be able to prepare his or her own food. I also want windows low enough to see out of from a wheelchair, a front-loading washer and dryer with the controls on the front, a spigot and small sink next to the stove for filling/emptying pans of water without having to travel with them. Perhaps there will be a "swing bar" gizmo to lift pots from sink to stove. I want front controls on the stove, too, with some kind of feature that would keep "little" hands out, but not limit access to a person with weaker hands or arms.

My master bath has a roll-in shower with nozzles in varying locations at varying heights.

A couple of things that have irked the crap out of me in all my house-planning research are (a) everyone says "modifications can be made," which means that, for $200 an hour, the architect will provide what should have been there in the first place; and (b) all plans I've seen so far that are designed for universal access look exactly the same! I guess they figure you're never going to have a party with fifteen or twenty guests or that your seven grandkids will never want to visit. If any of you remembers the Singing Nun, I'll quote her in regard to house plans available for accessibility today: "They all look ticky-tacky and they all look just the same."

I have also come up with plans for a device that would replace the old "sling-with-bare-ass-in-the-air" lift deal for the bathroom (or any other room, for that matter). I am talking to an engineer or two to see if we can't get this thing made and perhaps patented.

I guess it comes down to my absolute, written-in-stone belief that just because a person has a physical challenge, doesn't mean he or she doesn't have a life. They should be able to move easily through a simple, yet gracious home.

They should be able to sit and look out over a lake or a meadow or a city, without having to have six bodyguards named Bruno to get them there. They should be able to roast marshmallows over a campfire or drown a worm if they want to.

Helen Margo, what a wonderful house for anybody! You're brilliant! If you build it, I will come...and stay, and stay, and stay....

The Flutterbuds have dreamed, almost from the day we met each other, of co-owning a big, completely accessible house on lots of land, where MSers and their loved ones could gather to rest, relax, recreate, even reside. So, Margo, maybe you'd better add a few more bedrooms in your accessible loft! Don't be surprised if all of us show up with Helen on your dream doorstep one day. We'll officially name your house Fogbound Ranch!

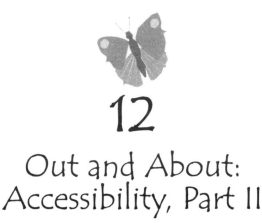

12

Out and About: Accessibility, Part II

Sharon Donna and I have decided to become defenders of good and fighters of evil. We plan to use our powers of MS and its resultant disabilities to kick the shit out of people who mess with disabled folk. We will have to be tied together with steel mesh to utilize our powers, though. Donna has a good left side; I have a good right. So, in order to kick ass, we'll have to be joined as one.

We thought Sally might draw a comic strip for us, since our powers do not include artistic ability. But we'll do the writing. We'll call it The MSHaps, and it will chronicle our MSadventures. Our arsenal already includes flying Depends® and a can of Whupass, which we'll carry into battle whenever we receive a call of dis(ability)tress.

Sal, we thought that, since we are comics, we could have awesome figures with gold and silver lamé costumes. I'd like opera-length gloves as well, a kind of Wonder Woman look.

Donna Yeah, Sal. I'd like to have good hair and long, metallic nails that light up when evil is being committed. It would help if our index fingers could be activated to point in the direction we need to go. We have MS and don't always recognize right and left, but we can normally follow a pointing finger. Shar, quit picking your nose with our directional indicator.

Sharon I wasn't picking my nose; I was scratching your eye, Donna. Now get down to business here. Anybody who has superhuman MS powers can help. Vickers, do you want to play? All your stored-up shit could be a lethal weapon.

Vicki We're going to use explosives?

Helen I want to play! Is it time for me to set up the factory for the plastique suppositories?

Donna Yes! I've been working on developing stupidity- and arrogance-seeking missiles. I visualize using a broad application for medical centers, legislatures, and insurance companies throughout the world, not to mention perfectly able-bodied people who park in handicapped spots.

Helen The world needs the MSHaps. I'm not sure the world is ready for us, but it needs us! Champions of MS, unite! By the way, what are we going to use for our identity signal? A Depends® silhouette across the night sky?

Sharon That's perfect! If we superimpose it across a full moon, it's even better.

Kim What can I do?

Sharon Maybe, since you're tiny and can fly and you have nursing experience, you could be the inserter of the plastique suppositories.

Kim Oh great. I am still sticking suppositories up old, cranky assholes. I've come a long way, baby!

Warning: Once this plan gets off the ground, anybody who blocks an MSer from going where she needs to go, doing what she needs to do, or getting what she needs to get will be dealt with appropriately. While Sharon and Donna organize the armory and design the costumes, though, we'll look for more immediate ways to get around the obstacles that we run into as soon as we leave our homes.

Dee I'm finding it harder and harder to spend any time at all away from home. I get confused and feel that I don't belong wherever I am. I think part of the reason for feeling "out of place" (even though nobody is making me feel that way) is that when I get out of my usual surroundings, I realize how disabled I have really become.

Me Isn't that the truth, Dee? I guess in our usual surroundings, we've adapted to the environment or have adapted the environment to suit our needs. We can go about our business without a second thought. We don't have to figure out how to get around barriers or follow a certain path (like from the bedroom to the bathroom—we're all used to that one!). But try to think about it and do it at the same time, and it's too much to handle at once. So the body shuts down one more time.

Janis I don't leave home very often. I always have to wait for somebody to take me anywhere. One of my best friends (the other half of my brain—she has MS, too) will take me to town tomorrow to go coat shopping. Neither of us goes into town very often, because we get too confused. So for both of us together, this should be quite the challenge!

For many of us, the inability to drive is the first barrier we encounter when we want to get out of the house. I stopped driving while I was in the middle of a *slam!* attack that took away most of the feeling and function in my feet. After I recovered (mostly) from that, I realized that my thought processes had slowed down so much that it wouldn't be safe for me to be in the driver's seat. I couldn't even remember how to stop my little scooter, so I didn't trust myself to find the brake pedal on a car. After ten years of hoping that I'd someday get back to "normal," then realizing I probably never would, I relinquished my license last year. Ron and my girls like to drive and don't mind acting as my chauffeurs, so it's usually not a problem. I've even talked myself into taking a cab a couple of times, even though Julie says, "There's no reason that my mom should have to take a cab!" (She said that just before she moved more than two hundred miles away.)

Most of us count on others for transportation, but some of our ladies fight to be able to continue driving. While Tara was still working (I mean outside your home, Tara!), she was able to get a completely adapted van through her state vocational rehabilitation agency. It has a dropped floor (to position her at the right height to drive from her power wheelchair), an automatic wheelchair lift, automatic door opener/closer, power wheelchair tiedown, electronic steering, and electronic gearshift. She asked her driving instructor, Paul St. Pierre, the director of Adaptive Driver Education at Crotched Mountain Rehabilitation Center in Greenfield, New Hampshire, to give us some pointers on selecting and using an adapted vehicle. Paul contributed enough information to fill a book in itself (I've encouraged him to write one!). There are different specifications for different needs, and combining the two for any individual is a very precise and complicated process. Paul said that his first, most important, bit of advice is, "Don't jump the gun!" He advises asking a doctor for a referral to a driver rehabilitation specialist, who can assess an MSer's current needs as well as take into account potential future needs and make adjustments to accommodate those, too. He said that Tara's van was customized to "compensate for weakness, conserve energy, prevent or reduce fatigue, maximize strengths, limit costs, and allow her to continue driving safely even if her condition deteriorates further." It's an expensive undertaking, so most folks would need assistance in carrying it out. Some of the references at the end of this book can provide connections to both local and national organizations that might be supportive.

For those who would be unable to drive no matter what adaptations are made, check with your local mass transit authority. Many provide special access services to disabled people, with pickup at the door and provisions for transporting wheelchairs.

What happens if you get where you want to go, either by driving yourself or riding with a driver, and you find that the only places to park are out in East Shoppers' Siberia? We realize that's often a dilemma for healthy people, too, but it's a particular concern when you're unable to walk any distance. We've had many discussions about the frustrations involved and have even come up with a few solutions to the problem.

Kathey The zoo in Omaha, Nebraska, is fantastic, one of the best ones I've ever been to (and believe me, I've been to a lot!). However, its parking is atrocious. There are probably more than five hundred spaces, and six of them are handicapped accessible ones. Six! I stopped at the guest services office and mentioned it. The lady there said they get a lot of complaints about it, so I asked her to pass mine along. I also wrote to the mayor of Omaha and to the director of the zoo. The answer I received? Something along the lines of, "We are following the ADA [Americans with Disabilities Act] regulations." I'm not sure we will be visiting that zoo again.

Me Kathey, if you ever do want to go back, or even if you don't, maybe you should challenge them on that statement. The ADA regulations are hard to decipher sometimes, and there are exceptions and exemptions for just about everything. But, in general, the guidelines say that 4 percent of parking places in lots should be accessible. So in a lot with five hundred spaces, there should have been at least twenty reserved for the handicapped. Maybe the persons who answered your letters (more than likely, a couple of secretaries rather than the mayor and the zoo director) weren't aware of the guidelines. Or, maybe the zoo really does have a valid reason not to provide the recommended number of spaces (I can't imagine what that would be). Or maybe they're all just blowing off your complaint, and they should be confronted about it. I heard an ADA specialist speak at an MS Society dinner recently, and she said that when somebody gives you "information" about accessibility compliance that isn't quite believable, you should ask to see documentation of the claim.

Kathey It's funny how my perspective on parking issues has changed. I remember a few years ago thinking, "Why are there so many disabled parking spots? If they'd have just one or two, the rest of us could park closer, too!" Now, of course, there never seems to be one available when I decide to "go fat butt" (I'm so glad Josh coined that phrase for me—he calls it a "fat butt" because he thought that little handicapped icon everywhere was a picture of somebody with a really fat butt sitting down. To this day, we still say, "Should we park in the fat butt today?").

Me Question: What has helped you the most in overcoming lack of accessibility? Answer: a handicapped placard and a fat butt!

Kathey Hey, it works for me. But, please, no pictures!

Robin That's the truth! Not about fat butts, Kathey; I mean about the handicapped spots. It's all about perspective and "walking" in the other guy's shoes. Of course, the handicapped places were always empty before, when you didn't need them. Now all of a sudden, there aren't any! It's a conspiracy, I tell you!

Me I'm surprised that more people who honestly need hand-icapped parking don't get permits for it. It's a simple matter of picking up a form from your local bureau of motor vehicles, then having the required evaluation, which may mean just getting a doctor's certification that you really have a disabling condition.

Dev The first time I applied for one, I was evaluated and told that I didn't need one yet. I was really glad they wouldn't give me one. Then, this past April my doctor insisted I get one. It was like somebody knocked the wind out of me. All I could think was that I'm getting worse. I just don't want to admit I really need it. After all, I look so good! But I'm going to have to either get the permit or give up shopping.

Helen You want to keep on looking so good, which involves being able to shop, right? So quit your stalling and go get the damned thing already!

Nadiza Your doctor is insisting on it because he wants you to keep your independence, Dev. The stress of having to walk a long way isn't good for you. Remember, less stress is better.

Margo I'm sending in my application for a permit as we speak. I'm actually kind of excited about it. For instance, at the trade show we did last weekend, I had to walk a long, long way to get into the building and then another good distance to our booth, with my hands full of stuff and using my cane besides. I could have used the placard then. But, on days that I don't feel I need it, I'm confident that I won't abuse the privilege. Maybe....

Kathey I still feel guilty parking in a spot for the "disabled" on my way into somewhere to spend the day walking around. I think I've used my placard probably four times and never when disabled parking is at a minimum.

Me Don't feel guilty, Kathey. That's part of the reason you have a placard—so that you don't wear yourself out walking from the parking lot to wherever you're supposed to be.

Joy Something else about having the permit: If I am ever stopped at a roadblock or involved in a fender bender, and it happens that I'm slurring my speech or staggering a bit, the cop might think I'm drunk. I can explain that I have MS and show him/her the placard as proof of a medical problem.

Dev I never thought of that. I have both problems at times. If I've been sitting and I stand up and start to walk, I kind of weave back and forth until I've been walking for a minute. Then I'm fine, but a police officer probably would think I was drunk. I'm glad you mentioned this.

Ramia I went to dinner one night with my kids, parked in a handicapped spot, and walked into the restaurant. Some man ripped into me: "What's wrong with you? Why are you parked there?" After I got over the shock, I thanked him for caring about those of us that need those spots. I told him I have MS and, although I don't appear to need the spot, I can't walk very far. He just kept shooting me dirty looks. I was seated, and I started to cry. Brian was so upset he wanted to go and yell at the man, "Can't you see how my mom had to walk to the table, using me or walls to balance?" The good thing that came out of it was that when we got home, Brian told me he was going to invent a robot that would go through my body and take all of that MS out. So keep your eyes open for Brian's cure.

Kathey I sure will, Ramia! I'm sorry you and the kids had to go through that, but I bet it was a learning experience for them. I'd say I hope the a–hole guy learned something too, but what are the chances of that?

Laura What annoys me is the folks who stop their vehicle at the curb or in the handicapped space for "just a few minutes." They think it's okay because they'll be leaving soon, or because they stay in the car. We have already pulled up to a spot, honked our horn, flashed the blue placard, and been ignored by the driver. My husband gets very angry. I just have him drop me off and park somewhere else. When I am alone, I don't have the guts to honk. If I can't find good parking, I either circle till I do, or I don't shop.

Here in New Jersey, in addition to your placard you get an ID card. To park in one of the accessible spots, the person carrying the card must be in the car. It's okay if you are being dropped off or picked up, as long as you are in the car on one side of the trip where it is parked in the spot.

Kathey Several nights in a row when I've gotten to work, there have been cars, with no placards or special plates, parked in the handicapped spots in the employees' lot. I know who these folks are. I've asked the security cops to ticket them, and they said they can't. So I talked to the nurse executive, and she spoke with the CEO, who happens to have a child who uses a wheelchair. He sent out a firmly worded memo to the security staff about calling the local PD to ticket these folks. It didn't work, as it happened again the other night. When I mentioned it to the cop, he said, "All I can do is put these little 'reminder' slips on their cars." This is at a hospital, for God's sake! I'll be talking to the nurse exec again today. I've made it my mission. Heck, I don't even park in the HP; why should someone else, just to "be closer"?

The guys at work who park there? They're mostly young, very healthy, just plain "I'm hot stuff, so I will park right here." I heard one of them say something about not looking for a parking place, because, "Why bother? The best ones are always empty."

Me Those poor maintenance guys! They're so physically

needy, how can you think about taking away their special parking privileges?

Kathey I know; I'm just a bitch. Unfeeling, uncaring. But they "look so good." No, wait, they don't.

Nadiza The night crew at our grocery store always parked in the handicapped parking spaces. When they worked past the opening time of the store, that meant there were no handicapped spaces available. I complained at the customer service desk and was told that the night crew did this for their safety. I told them that they needed to either move the cars by the time the store opens or not park there. Again, they said that it was for safety. I told them that parking their cars one space over was not going to put the night crew or their cars in extra danger. I then informed them that if the crew insisted on parking illegally, I would not only call the police, but I would also spread the word that the store did not care about handicapped customers. I haven't seen them parked there since.

Kathey I've been using those "tickets" that say, "You are parked in a spot reserved for the disabled. I will trade you my disability for your parking space." I keep a stack of them in my glove box and just stick one under the windshield wiper of illegally parked cars.

Nadiza I would prefer a big sign that lets all passersby know that the person is parked in the wrong spot. Do you think flashing lights would be too much?

Kathey Heck, flashing lights, a siren, and a PA system wouldn't be too much. I don't mean folks who "should" have a tag and don't (you know, people who park there because of how they are feeling—that's illegal, too, but not so bad). I've noticed, too, how horridly inconvenient some of the special parking places are. That's not a problem for me right now, but for folks who have to slog through traffic and up curbs in snow and rain with a wheelchair? Not good. I've gotten two businesses in my little town to change the location of their spaces.

▲▲▲

So we manage to get from the parking lots into the businesses themselves. Then what?

▲▲▲

Robin I have been in WalMart and used the scooters they so kindly provide. But the baskets attached to them aren't big enough to hold more than a couple of small items. When I go to the grocery, they have wheelchairs, but how can you shop from a wheelchair and push a cart at the same time?

Kim I go with my crutches instead of my wheelchair, then get a shopping cart, use that for support, and put my crutches inside it, off to the side. My fear is the shopping malls. They don't usually have carts, so walking with crutches and carrying packages from store to store is impossible.

Robin I can't remember the last time I "strolled" the mall, for this reason. I don't dare go shopping unless it's in one store, just in and out. I take my cane, too. If nothing else, it proves I'm not drunk! This type of thing makes me seriously consider getting a scooter.

Helen <sigh> I use the shopping cart for support instead of a walker or cane. But malls, especially, are hard for me. Each store may have a shopping cart, but then you have to go from store to store. Without a scooter, it's hard, and with one, the aisles are too narrow. The thing that bugs me is that many stores don't have enough room between displays for a scooter. If I have my scooter, I have to get out of it to look at some things, and it's a real pain in the ass.

Vicki This is where we differ. In mall stores, I seldom get off my scooter. If the aisles are too narrow for my scooter, I go through anyway. If there are clothes on racks that get in my way, they get dirty. I figure if the stores aren't concerned about handicapped needs, I'm not concerned about getting their clothes dirty.

Helen Yeah, but I'm so short, if I try to force my way through, I get hit in the face by sleeves hanging off hangers.

Donna A football helmet would take care of this and help you maintain anonymity at the same time.

Vicki No helmets! If you wear a helmet, the sleeves can't clean the cinnamon roll icing off your lips!

Laura Many stores just don't care about wheelchairs, walkers, or strollers. The people using them are a small segment of the population and tend to not have as much disposable income. The stores feel they can make more money by having extra displays out than they will lose from a couple of handicapped people not being able to shop there.

Joy From a business standpoint, it makes sense to cater to the majority of your customers and potential customers, and that means offering as large a selection of merchandise as possible in the amount of space they have. Personally, I can shrug this off, because I do most of my shopping from catalogs, television, or online. I have to pay shipping costs, but this is offset by the fact that I avoid impulse shopping and consider each purchase more carefully. Also, sales tax is usually avoided, not to mention the stress of driving, parking, fighting the crowds, standing in checkout lines, risking being mugged, etc.

Me Joy, I've been doing much of my shopping by mail or online. Last year I got an offer for free shipping and handling on one order. I ordered some things and wrote a note to the company saying that I appreciated not having to pay shipping charges since I often have to rely on catalog shopping. I guess those companies really do info-share about their customers, because all of a sudden I started getting offers from lots of other places for free shipping. It really paid to speak up!

Kathey But when you shop like that, you don't get to go ogle the cute guys at the mall! Smart management folks (and, yes, I've heard they do exist, somewhere) know that for every complaint they get, in writing or otherwise, there are a hundred people that wanted to complain but didn't. That's why it's so important to speak up on this stuff. After all, how do you think disabled parking spots got there in the first place? Somebody complained loudly enough. Maybe my complaint will make a difference someday to somebody.

Dev Sunday I went shopping and decided not to use a cane. I was walking around the store, looking, but not touching anything. After a while, I noticed this man following me. He kept walking slowly by me and staring. One time he almost knocked me down. When I looked at the tag on his shirt, I noticed he worked for the store. I finally gave up and went to find Mike in the store. When we got outside, I told Mike about it. He said, "He probably thought you were drunk. Why didn't you tell me while we were in the store?" I felt awful! I would rather the guy thought I was shoplifting than drunk. I almost went to the office to report him, but I didn't because I'm so paranoid about the way I walk. I didn't want to draw attention to myself. I really wish I'd said something, but I didn't know what to think or say at the time. I know it's not the man's fault. Now that I think about it, he did look awfully funny flitting around, staring at me. He was a pretty big guy, and when he almost knocked me down, all I could think about was getting the hell out of there before I fell. I know one thing; I will not go in a store without that cane again. Even if I don't need it that day, it's going with me.

Joy   I think if that happened to me (and now that it's happened to you, I'll be mentally prepared for it), once I identified him as a store employee, I would have looked him in the face and said, "I'm not high on anything. I have MS and today is a wobbly day," or something like that.

Me   Go back, Dev! It's not too late to let the store manager know that one of the employees made you very uncomfortable. Let us know what happens.

Dev [the next day]   There's not really a lot to tell, Judy Lynn. I just wish I'd done it sooner. I went back to the store and asked to talk to the manager. I told him that I have MS and that I was embarrassed because one of the employees seemed to be following me around the store because he thought I was drunk. At first he was kind of snotty and told me that they have no way of knowing what condition their customers are in. I said, "Why didn't he just ask?" and he said that would be an invasion of my privacy. I asked what he thought following me all over the store, running around me, and almost causing me to fall is. I showed him who the guy was, and the jerk denied the whole thing. I guess the manager could tell he was lying. He apologized profusely, made the guy apologize, too, and offered me a gift certificate. I told him to keep it and give it to the next customer they humiliate, because I won't be shopping in their store anymore. I feel a helluva lot better!

Margo   I saw something scary one day when I was shopping. A woman had a seizure, and the clerks were desperately trying to move all those damned racks so the paramedics could get to the woman to treat her. I'd like to say I passed by politely holding my tongue, but I didn't. I told the clerk that their racks were too cram-packed in there and what a hazard they presented by blocking off the elevator. She snapped back, "The lady had a seizure!" Yes, she did, and wasn't it a shame that her medical assistance was hampered by the racks and racks of clothing crammed so closely together? Then, after they got all the flippin' racks moved so the paramedics could get their gear in from the aisle, the clerks had to move them again to clear the mythical path to the elevator so the medics could get the woman out. I've never forgotten it, and I still wish I'd written a letter to the store manager and the fire marshal.

Robin It's interesting that you bring this up today because of what just happened to me. Yesterday there was a fire drill for the tower that I work in. Well, guess which floor I'm on? The eighth! Oh, yeah, the elevators? They're turned off. I just looked at my coworker and said that there was no way in hell I'd be able to walk down eight flights of stairs. I guess if there were a real fire, I'd make myself do it. But for a drill? Nope.

I put myself in my boss's office and shut the door. My coworker came back later and told me that she'd spoken to the fireman, and asked what they do if there's a wheelchair user. She found out that in those cases, the fire marshals should be told who the people are that can't do stairs, and they get taken down via the service elevator. So that's something new that I learned: talk to someone in a building with elevators to find out what the procedure is for somebody who can't do stairs. Sheesh! I never even thought about that until this happened.

Kathey I imagine that in the middle of an evacuation would not be the time to say, "Oh, by the way...."

Laura We have people assigned to make sure the handicapped get out of our office okay. I told them not to bother to assign somebody to me. I'd rather just get myself out. We have one guy there who can't walk at all. The person who was assigned to him was outside smoking during the last evacuation.

Kathey While we're sort of on the subject, remember I told

you all that I was upset that the Oklahoma City Zoo didn't have any scooters for rent? I had a great talk with the guest services director yesterday. She said they didn't have scooters because they didn't want to worry about someone rolling out of control down one of the big hills there. I told her that the newer scooters don't roll; they only move when the motor turns the wheels. I mentioned a couple of places I've been to that she should call and ask for recommendations about brands. She was going to call around today and said that by the time I returned to their zoo, they would have them!

Me Way to go, Kathey! I know you travel a lot, and you collect travel brochures—is there lots of information available on whether or not places that you plan to visit are accessible?

Kathey Very much so. Most brochures for major tourist attractions and for hotels/motels use that adorable little symbol for places that are wheelchair-friendly. Some go into greater detail about accessibility accommodations. If they don't, most places (even tiny ones) have 800 numbers where you can get the information. Most places I enjoy are nature/outdoor-type things. Often the brochures will say something like "parts of the park, area, what have you, are not handicapped accessible." That at least it gives me a clue about what kind of stairs, etc., may be involved.

Along with the brochure thing, I've been pleasantly surprised at the amount of information available on the Internet about tourist spots. Even the tiniest places seem to have a website now. With a click of the button, you can send an e-mail that says, "I'd like to know about the physical layout of your facility." Sometimes you even get an answer!

Laura I just read that Disney World is having a hard time with healthy people renting wheelchairs and using them because, if you're in one, you get line preference.

193

Kathey   Josh told me about this when he was at Disney
World two years ago. A whole, big family (ten or twelve of
them) would take turns riding in the wheelchair and getting
moved to the front of the lines! Josh and his friends tried to
tell an employee but weren't taken seriously (because they
were kids?). Of course, if it happened now, I would call
Disney and raise a ruckus. Two years ago I just thought, "It's
lousy that they got away with that." Again, isn't it funny how
much difference a couple of years (and a few MouSe poopies
in your brain) can make?

I'm going to end this chapter on a triumphant, "good news"
note. Anybody who has known me for ten minutes (if I can
manage to stay quiet about it for even that long) is aware that I'm
a great Neil Diamond fan(atic). My friend Donna and I have
attended as many of his local concerts as possible during the past
twenty-five years. Last fall I saw that Neil was scheduled to do a
concert at FirStar Center (the coliseum-type arena in Cincinnati)
in December. The minute the tickets went on sale, I was online
to a ticket agency to order them. I clicked the little "fat butt" logo
on the website and filled in the information requesting wheelchair accessible seating. When the order confirmation arrived, I
checked with the agency to make sure the seats were accessible; I
received an e-mail note: "These seats are not accessible." Period.
No explanation, even after I sent another e-mail asking, in effect,
"Why the hell not?"

So I contacted the agency by phone. The young lady I spoke
with tried to be helpful (she kept going to her supervisor to find
answers to my questions) but wasn't able to come up with an
acceptable resolution. I was told that I could exchange my tickets
for ones in the wheelchair seating area, up in nosebleed heaven.
If I wanted to enter the facility in my wheelchair and go on
crutches to a regular seat, I'd have to buy an extra ticket, rent

space, in effect, to leave the chair in the handicapped section. According to the information the agent had, "fire regulations prohibit wheelchairs anyplace in the arena except for the designated area." I moaned and groaned and got mad and then decided to let the whole deal ride as it was, thinking I'd find some way to get to my seat.

Then a MonStrous attack hit and kept me in the wheelchair for most of the next month, including the time of the concert. If the star had been anybody else, I would have dropped the whole idea and stayed home. But this was Neil Diamond, and this was one thing that I swore the MonSter wouldn't make me give up.

I sent an e-mail to FirStar Center, described the events to date, quoted ADA specifications that the venue seemed to be violating, and asked if any resolution was possible. I received a prompt answer from Jenny, the director of Box Office Operations at FirStar Center. She told me that the ticket agency's computers weren't set up to assign accessible seating via the Internet and that all the information I'd received through its sources was wrong. Jenny said that at FirStar Center, they were willing to do "anything" to make sure that disabled persons could safely and comfortably patronize events at their facility. She more than proved it! She issued new tickets for accessible seats for Donna and me. She made arrangements for me to store my wheelchair in the hockey penalty boxes a couple of feet from our seats. She greeted us personally when we arrived and made sure a security guard was available all evening in case I wanted to retrieve my wheelchair or needed other assistance. In other words, the staff of the center treated us like royalty. It was one of the best evenings of my life! Donna and I sat in the front row, just a few feet from the stage, way down at the bottom of the arena. But I felt like I was living far above anything that MS could do to me.

The moral of the story? Sometimes accessibility is there, but we don't have easy access to that information. So, if you have a complaint or concern about getting into or getting around in any public place, go directly to somebody in a managerial position at the place. In all likelihood, that person can either give you the correct information and make accommodations or start the ball rolling to get the facility to comply with ADA guidelines. Then go and have a great time!

And join me in a hearty "Ha!" to the MonSter. Maybe we don't need the MSHaps after all.

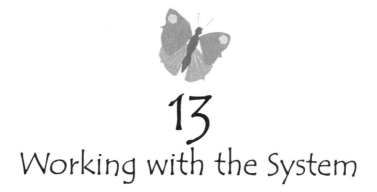

13
Working with the System

Kathey Okay, here goes Kath. Hang on, ladies! A year ago, before MS showed up, I was working eighty-four hours every two weeks; now I'm working fewer than sixty-four. I've had to cut back in order to be able to function at all, both at work and away from it. I have fantastic insurance but still spend big bucks on co-pays for meds (I know, I shouldn't whine. At least I can get them and have insurance to cover the rest of the cost), plus $10 per visit at the doctor or physical therapist or whatever. I had to go out and get a new truck, so vehicle payments doubled, as did insurance. Utilities are through the roof (although I hardly ever turned on the air conditioner in the house. All those cold showers, courtesy of being separated from Kirk so much, helped there!).

I haven't paid last month's mortgage yet; I don't have the money. My truck payment is due Tuesday. I have shut-off notices from the gas, electricity, and water companies. The house is falling apart.

I have no credit, no savings, no backup for emergencies. Who needed it? I was young and healthy, with a great career ahead of me. Ptooooie! And, I'm one of the lucky ones! I have a good job. I have good insurance. I live in my own nice (okay, messy) house. I drive a new truck.

But, if my mind keeps melting, and my body keeps falling to pieces, what then? I have no family to fall back on. It's me and Josh. He *depends* on me. I can apply for Social Security Disability Income and long-term disability from work (if they allow me to reenroll since I dropped the coverage last year). But how do I make it through the six-month waiting period (and that's an optimistic estimate—heck, SSDI could take six *years*)? So I start saving money, right? Yeah, right. I can save pennies, until I am out of gas and have to get to work, then into rolls they go.

It totally sucks that this damned disease just takes *everything*: intelligence, mobility, continence, independence, *money*.

I'm not really whining, I swear to God; I'm happy in so many ways. I'm just being realistic. And I'm quite a bit frightened. I hear you have to hit bottom sometimes before you can start going up. I figure that should happen right about now.

Sally Kathey, I hear you. The problems are there, but I don't know how to fix them. I've just pulled in my horns and decided that I would get by on what I have, but it isn't easy. I had to give up driving, not because I can't drive, but because I don't have the money to fix the car and renew the registration—so it rots in the garage. I am fortunate that the only person that depends on me is my dog, and she doesn't care if I wear rags or if we live in "welfare housing." I hope she doesn't notice the mismatched furniture. There have been times when I chose between food for me and food for her. Guess who won! Still, I am basically a happy person and have learned to look for my joys in different places than I did before. Thank the goddesses I found you folks!

I almost feel guilty. I'm more than adequately fed and housed. Thanks to Ron's good job with good insurance, most of my medicines, office visits, and medical supplies are at least partly paid for. I have a devoted husband, two generous daughters, and lots of other family and friends who take me where I need to go (no worries about how to personally finance cars, insurance, and gas). I can't think of anything that I need but that is denied to me because I have MS. I've wondered occasionally what kind of hardships I'd encounter if Ron or my girls were ever taken from my life. Other than that, I've rarely thought beyond my own self-satisfied existence. I'm learning to not be so complacent, after paying a bit more attention to the struggles that some MSers go through.

Helen I'd like to address some concerns of those of us who, like Kathey [and Kim, Sally, Bren, Tara, and Jamie], are considered by mainstream society to be "single." This includes the gay and lesbian community, people who are cohabiting without marriage, and those who are without partners either by choice or by chance. Our society is oriented toward the heterosexual marriage module. The concept of "family values," as it is frequently called in political rhetoric, is aimed at the nuclear family. That's the one that lives in the suburbs, with two spouses, one and four-fifths children, a minivan and a car, and a dog. The gay, lesbian, or otherwise unmarried couple, who might also own a house, be raising children, have a minivan and a dog, and who may have been together for many years, still are considered single.

My partner, Janni, and I have been together for seventeen years. This is as long as, or longer than, many of our legally married, heterosexual friends and relatives have been together. However, Janni cannot claim me on her insurance, we cannot file taxes jointly, and were it not for each of us having the other's power of attorney, we would have no say about jointly owned property, long-term medical care, or any other legal or financial matter that might impact our lives.

Neither of us can receive Social Security death benefits through the other, nor can the income or circumstances of either of us be considered in calculating disability or retirement benefits for the other. I cannot get health insurance on my own to pay for medication, dental care, hearing tests, or hearing aids, all of which I could receive from Janni's insurance if our relationship were legally recognized.

The gay and lesbian population is estimated to be between 5 and 10 percent of the adult population at large. Any other ethnic, racial, or religious minority group of this size, denied benefits simply because it didn't fit into the traditional mold, would have started a revolution by now.

Me Helen, maybe it's time to start one. Since shortly after I "met" you online, I've known that you're lesbian and that you and Janni are in a committed relationship. I never gave it a second thought, except maybe to congratulate myself for being liberal enough to not judge your lifestyle. All of that time, I've watched you struggle (and never quite succeed) to get adequate medical and dental care, reliable transportation, and all the other essentials that I take for granted. I never considered that being disabled *and* being single (gay/unmarried by choice or circumstance) could join forces to become one, huge, insurmountable handicap. I'm appalled by my own lack of knowledge about resources that you, or any other unmarried MSers, could tap into, in order to find the kinds of help that are built into the marriage contract. I promise that if there's ever a chance for laws to be passed that will eradicate this form of discrimination, I'm going to get off my smug butt and vote for them. Maybe your words here will filter through the minds of everybody who reads them and help us, as a system within a society, to reconsider the existing laws and attitudes. I thank you for opening my eyes just a little bit, Helen.

▲▲▲

In the meantime, we can talk about some of the facts we've uncovered and the experiences we've had as we've accessed existing resources to ease the financial burdens that the MonSter imposes. Once a person is unable to work, the obvious course of action is to apply for Social Security Disability Income and/or other long-term disability benefits. As Kathey mentioned, it can take six months to several years to start collecting payments. So it's imperative, especially if there isn't another wage earner in the family, to come as close as possible to meeting the eligibility requirements before actually leaving employment. That will lessen the chances of having to go through a protracted period with no income at all. Each case is judged independently (one person's inability to perform her work duties may be deemed inconsequential for another person, depending on education, training, experience, and the availability of work in the person's field). There's no way to determine ahead of time that the Social Security Administration will agree that any one person qualifies as "disabled." In general, an applicant must have an impairment that has lasted, or is expected to last, for at least twelve continuous months. That impairment must have prevented the person from "engaging in substantial gainful activity" during that time. This can be kind of touchy for MSers in the remitting/relapsing stage or type of MS. If symptoms subside after eleven months and twenty-nine days, the person still has MS but isn't eligible for disability benefits. I was able to hold off for fifteen years after my diagnosis before I applied for SSDI. By that time, there wasn't much doubt that the MonSter was going to hang around for longer than a year.

The next step, after an MSer concludes that she'll meet the requirements, is to contact the Social Security Administration to obtain the application forms and instructions on how to fill them out. (Check the resources section in the back of this book for toll-free numbers and web addresses for information and forms.) Then it's time to gather evidence, fill out the paperwork, go through a phone interview with an SSA agent, and possibly have more medical tests ordered by SSA. That's followed by a waiting period: six months from the last date you were able to work, if SSA says you're eligible right away; otherwise, it's however long it takes to convince SSA that you truly can't earn an income.

Of course, all of this is based on the premise that a person worked and paid Social Security taxes long enough to qualify for benefits. Anybody who becomes disabled before she has enough time invested can check into receiving SSI, which can be received on disability even if the person never contributed to Social Security. It isn't much, but every little bit helps!

Chris When I applied (for SSDI—I'd worked under Social Security for more than twenty years!), I got as much information as I could from people who had already applied, so I knew what to expect. I gathered all my doctors' records to send. I made sure that, in my answers on the form, I came across as doing as little as possible so they wouldn't think I can do more than I really can! I didn't offer any information other than what was asked for on the form and didn't go into a lot of detail. I kept copies of everything that I sent them, too, so I'd have them if my approval didn't go through. I must have done it right, since I was approved the first time!!!

Me I agree that you shouldn't leave any openings for SSA to overestimate your capabilities, Chris. But I did offer more information than they asked for, at least as far as describing the medical problems that kept me from working. At the time, fatigue wasn't a valid consideration for eligibility, but I told them about mine. I don't think they asked about bladder control problems, either, but they heard about it from me. When they asked how I spent my days, I went through every hour, making sure I mentioned the times that I have to stop what I'm doing and rest. Then I added another description of the days when I can't do much of anything but rest. I guess they got tired of reading everything I wrote, because they approved it on the first try.

Kim   I got it the first time, also. And I did the same thing. I told every single detail. I think I added a page and a half about what my day was like. I told them about my naps, my pain; you name it, they heard about it!

Dee   When I applied for SSDI, I was told to answer the questions as I would on one of my worst days. I had worked with SSA in my job as a social worker, so I knew that one needs to carefully consider the answer to each question. Why are they asking it? What will it tell them? Such as: What kind of hobbies do you have? If I tell them that I enjoy using the computer, they might assume that I could use a computer in a job. Yes, I do enjoy the computer and I can use one. But I also know that my eyes get blurry, my fingers begin to have trouble with the keys, my right arm gets weaker, etc., when I use one. I certainly could not work on one for eight hours every day! So, you have to think every response through completely, while remaining truthful.

Bunny   I was denied the first time, so I hired an attorney. I didn't have the energy to play Social Security's games. I was denied again and then went in front of a judge. I did finally get SSDI, but it was not granted because of MS symptoms. They geared their decision to the psychological aspect of my disability. In other words, even the SSA thinks it's all in my head!

Me   I was relieved that I didn't have to hire an attorney. It already makes me angry that disabled people have to wait a minimum of six months for benefits after a zillion doctors certify that they have a chronic, incurable disease. Let's say that SSA denies an MSer's claim. So she (okay, I realize this is pertinent to men also, but this is just one example) waits half an eternity to have an appeal heard and finally hires a lawyer to fight for approval. Meanwhile, all the benefits that should have started paying out at the end of that first six months have been accruing (without interest, I might add!). The attorney steps in, presents the same evidence that the MSer already submitted. The judge finally gives approval, which, after all that time, most likely would have happened even without the intervention of an attorney. Then the attorney pockets a huge percentage of the money that the MSer should have gotten months earlier.

Dee I know that the idea of hiring a lawyer is controversial. It's true that some folks get their benefits without one. After my claim was denied the first time, I went ahead with a lawyer. I couldn't think clearly enough about how to answer any more questions, and I thought I had a better chance if an attorney helped me fill out the paperwork.

The MS Society has a workbook on SSDI that I found very helpful, also. I'm sure that most chapters have copies in their libraries and will lend them to you. Of course, I received a lot of helpful suggestions from my sisters here online, as well as in the chats.

I also kept copies of every report I had sent. If I had to go through it again, I didn't want to contradict myself.

▲▲▲

If you have minor children, they're also entitled to Social Security benefits at the time that your eligibility is approved. That's true even if you have been working only to pay off your classic Volkswagen Beetle or to add to your collection of Beatles memorabilia. I wasn't working for either of those goals but missed out on getting benefits for my girls. I applied for SSDI a few months after Julie turned eighteen. Luckily, though, that was also the time that she was ready to enter college. Although we'd already secured what we thought was maximum financial aid for her, I contacted her college and told them I'd had to stop working. The change in our income actually made a difference, and they increased her grants!

Vicki When I talked to the SSDI agent this morning, I was told that the kids will receive a pittance in addition to what I receive. By the time they turn eighteen, they should have a decent college fund in the bank.

Janis I talked to somebody at the Social Security office about my kids. It turns out that they will receive back pay for the past two years! It's about time! The lady said that there was a note attached to my file to contact me about getting the kids signed up, but, unfortunately, nobody followed through with it. She said she was glad that I finally contacted them, since it should have been taken care of along with my application.

At the same time that a disabled person applies for SSDI, it's wise to find out if an employer has been paying premiums or deducting payments from salary for long-term disability insurance. If that's true, then apply for that concurrently with the application for SSDI. It's a lot easier to make two copies of every record, or write in the same answer twice to a question, than it is to go back later and start from scratch.

Vicki This morning (early!) I had my phone interview for long-term disability benefits. I couldn't have talked to a nicer man. I have a feeling this is going to work out without too many hassles. If I fill out the application form in purple ink, that should help, right? [Purple is the Froup's "signature" color.]

Me You remembered to change out of that torn nightgown before the interviewer called, didn't you, Vicki?

Vicki Well, no. I thought it would be *better* if I looked like a bag lady.

I got my copy of the form that my employer filled out. It states that there is no type of work that I can do for them with the restrictions I have. It looks like an approval just waiting to happen for me!

Meanwhile, we wait for SSDI approval, too.

Which reminds me, is SSDI taxable? I don't think it is, but I'm not an accountant, nor do I pretend to be one.

Me You don't even play one on TV, do you? Anyway, SSDI sure is taxable, Vickers, sorry to say. That bugs the hell out of me, because, at least in the beginning of getting benefits, you end up paying taxes on money that you'd already paid taxes on when you earned it.

Helen No it's not, unless you get more than twenty thousand dollars a year between that and any other pensions, which is time to look for snowballs in hell....

Me You're kidding, Helen! If that's true, then I'm going to be double-pissed. Every time I've figured our tax returns, it has worked out that I have to pay taxes on all of my LTD payments and almost all of my SSDI payments. I'm going to go check the tax book right now....

Dee Doesn't it depend on how much you make? I don't think SSDI is taxable by itself.

Me Okay, I'm no more pissed now than I was to start with. I just checked the *Complete Idiot's Guide* and my previous returns. The system still stinks, but we've been doing it right.

SSI benefits aren't taxable; SS retirement and disability benefits are, following the IRS formula. If you're married and filing jointly, you have to pay if your combined income is more than thirty-two thousand dollars. If you're married and filing separately, and you lived with your spouse for even one day during the year, your benefits are taxable no matter how much either spouse made. That said and done, you have to go through a whole big formula of computations (which I just let my tax program calculate). It ends up that you have to pick the lesser of two numbers that result from all of that math. For Ron and me, the lesser is 85 percent of total Social Security benefits. That's how much we have to pay taxes on, in addition to all other taxable income. This is all based on one spouse collecting Social Security and the other or both having earned income. I'm not sure how it would work if both were on SS and neither had other income. I guess it wouldn't be taxable in that case.

Anybody who got waylaid with us into this little tax maze, remember that I'm not a qualified guide through the IRS's labyrinth. Please ask an accountant, or check updated rules from the Internal Revenue Service each year to determine which disability benefits are taxable.

Kathey How about insurance if/when I have to quit working? I whine about co-pays now; I can't imagine paying full price for these drugs. It would cost close to $2,000, just for what I'm on now.

Me Kathey, if that day comes, check into an interim "catastrophic coverage" policy. Karen and Julie have both used those during times when they were between jobs or working at places that didn't offer medical benefits. These are usually inexpensive and don't require medical exams ahead of time. They're intended mostly to pick up extraordinary costs, like emergency surgery. The deductibles are monumental before they start paying for doctor visits or drugs. But for somebody like you, the deductibles would be met in a very short time (without having to resort to having surgery to meet them!).

Once you qualify for SSDI, you have a waiting period of two years before Medicare automatically kicks in. There's no premium for Part A, hospital coverage. You can pay a premium to receive Part B, medical coverage. Most people find that insufficient to cover their needs; there are now Medicare-affiliated, private managed-care plans (available at a somewhat higher premium) that provide more comprehensive coverage for doctor visits and drugs.

MSers who don't qualify for SSDI might still be able to get medical coverage (Medicaid), as Bren found out.

Bren Medical insurance for me? Well, y'all know *that* story. No company will cover me, at least not at a rate I can afford. Or they won't cover the MS, or they won't cover the MS for the first twelve-to-eighteen months. So, I talked to my former social worker the other day. She said I might qualify for Medicaid. I told her that I'd looked into that before and was told that if I'm not eligible for disability benefits, then it's a "no go." She said, "Not the Medicaid you get because of disability, but the one you get because of low income." Of course, I perked right up. So I'm going to apply for it. That would be a lifesaver!

Sally Here in California, some people who are on SSDI can get Medicaid (which covers more than Medicare) if they pay a certain amount each month. It's based on the difference between the SSDI benefit received and the current SSI amount. At least it is good for those expensive emergency situations or expensive medications. I think this is one of the few things that California has that's better than the other states!

Kim That is great, Sally! Here we can't get medical coverage at all without being damned near homeless. I still can't believe that they don't consider *rent* an expense here. It sucks! The Medicaid office said that I'd have to pay about five grand out of pocket before they would cover my bills. Well, like I can afford that much! It kind of makes me wish I hadn't received SSDI approval. At least then (on Medicaid), I could afford my freaking meds and the occasional trip to the doctor when needed!

Then Helen told us about applying for government-funded medical assistance.

Helen Well, I got it, all right, but they consider that I have $105 a month "excess" income, out of my big whoop $709! So I have to do a $631 spend-down in the next six months to get any help for the rest of the year. The system sure is shitty!

Me How in the world did they come up with that figure? Is it supposed to be a percentage of your yearly income?

Helen It's actually $105 per month, not $631 annually. They review it in six months, but so far they have decided I have $105 too much income per month, so I have to pay the first $631 out of pocket.

Vicki Just exactly what is it you do with that extra money each month, Ms. Helen? If you didn't waste money on food, you'd be able to pay your own medical expenses. Geez!

Me You didn't put on your application that you got a vet to do Chance's [Helen's crippled dog] surgery gratis, did you?

Helen I may be dumb, but I ain't ignorant! They'd tell me that if I can afford medical care for my dog, I don't need their help!

Bren Another option I have, if the Medicaid thing doesn't work out, is to contact Vocational Rehab. Perhaps they'll help me get a job I can actually do, and that has benefits!

Bren reported shortly afterwards that the State Bureau of Vocational Rehabilitation at least got her started toward her goal.

Bren I got all of my study materials and supplies for the schooling that Voc. Rehab. arranged for me. If this works out, I'll be a medical transcriptionist someday soon! I can study at home, as I'm able to do it. They're even willing to help me find a job, preferably one that I can do from home, after I finish the courses!

Donna The Powers That Be were looking out for me when I called Arkansas Rehab. Services a couple of weeks ago for an appointment. The caseworker assigned to me, Shed, is an old friend from my intern days in juvenile court. Shed said he's certain I will be accepted. He said that with the MS and the other problems I've had (maybe all this crap is an asset after all!), I fit neatly into all three categories used to determine eligibility. Once I'm accepted into the program, they will regularly evaluate my needs and provide equipment and assistance to keep me working.

I didn't expect so much positive energy from the

beginning. Shed and I discussed more coping skills and confidence builders. He made out a list of confidence builders for me to include in my self-talk. If I'm half as good as he says, I'm good! We also made a list of what I consider my negatives and ways to either work through them and turn them into positives or to neutralize them.

In the meantime, I'd sure appreciate prayers and good thoughts on this. If I'm lucky, I'll be disabled enough to meet the requirements but healthy enough to be a good risk to be included in the program.

[The "positive energy" worked for Donna. A few months later, she went back to work in a civilian position at her beloved police department!]

Sharon This is wonderful! It was a smart move for you to get in touch with the rehabilitation services office. I made it through an MS attack while working, and vocational rehab. saw me through the adaptations necessary. New Hampshire Vocational Rehab. will bend over backwards to keep you employed.

Tara New Hampshire does more than that! Besides the help I've gotten from the Vocational Rehab. bureau, I've had homemakers, help with paying bills, and lots of other services. When I had surgery, there were nurses provided, home health aides to help me shower and dress, companions to fix meals, physical therapists, occupational therapists; I was inundated with help! And I welcomed it with open arms. [Some of Tara's other experiences with NH Vocational Rehab. are cited in Chapter 11, "Up, or at Least Around."]

Robin Connecticut's Bureau of Rehabilitative Services, which, I think, is New Hampshire's twin agency, helped me to replace my hearing aids a couple of years ago. I didn't know the agency even existed until somebody told me while I was shopping for the hearing aids. So I applied, I qualified, and they replaced them. Now I know that they'll be able to help me with the MS, too, if I need it. Last spring, our local NMSS chapter had a seminar that included people from the BRS who talked about the resources available through them.

When assistance from the "system" isn't available or doesn't quite make up for a financial deficit, there's always the chance that approaching somebody with authority to offer "a break" can help.

Bren Yesterday, when I got my prescriptions filled, my wonderful pharmacist crossed out my co-pay amount on the bill, and said "You know we don't have to charge this, don't you?" So, for now, I don't even have to make a co-payment for the medications I'm getting.

Kathey I can't afford the huge payments on my truck anymore. I'm having trouble driving it, too. The clutch/shift coordination is more than I can handle, and my eye troubles make parking it tough. On Monday, I'll be going to the local Ford dealer to drop off my truck and pick up my new little car (with an automatic transmission)!

Me That's great, Kath! The truck lease seemed to be an irrevocable commitment when you talked about it before. How did you manage to get that settled?

Kathey A phone call to the CEO of Ford Motor Credit, with mention of a few names, like the local director of the NMSS and the lead counsel for the Missouri Governor's Office for Disability Advocacy helped, I think!

Kathey's mention of the National Multiple Sclerosis Society reminds me—any MSer who is in need of assistance of any kind should contact his or her local chapter of the NMSS. Some chapters have funds set up to help clients through almost any kind of emergency. Even if they can't offer direct assistance, they're likely to have commitments from local businesses, organizations, and agencies willing to cooperate in helping people with MS.

Whatever the need, there is help available somewhere, either in the "system" or in the goodness (and common sense) of other human beings. It doesn't hurt to ask for it!

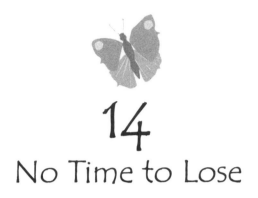

14

No Time to Lose

Tara I feel like I have been given such a gift, with all the time I have now. I get up with no plans whatsoever each and every day. I think, what am I going to play with today? I absolutely love every day! I fill it with drawing, painting, writing, sculpting, making medicine bags, embroidering, and so much more! I feel like an adult who has been given a second chance at childhood. I play and play and never run out of days for it!

If I had read Tara's note a few years ago, I would have presumed that she was an incredible idealist, hopelessly out of touch with reality. At that time, I was still trying to adjust to the fact that I'm not able to work outside my home any longer. I was convinced I'd never again have a purpose in life, that I would just sit here with the MonSter for the next however-many years and wait for some justification for my existence to fall into my lap. I wouldn't have believed that a fellow MSer could actually sing the praises of joblessness.

Now, though, I can read it and remember that less than three years ago, Tara was one of the many Flutterbuds (myself included) who were either struggling to stay employed or mourning the recent loss of a career. I remember that those of us who had to give up working found ourselves with too many of those empty hours we'd actually prayed for such a short time before. I recall watching (and participating) as, one by one, we faced feelings of helplessness, worthlessness, nothingness. We talked about nearly suffocating in boredom and boredom-induced fatigue. Then, gradually or suddenly, we each discovered new interests and skills or refined old ones to accommodate our changing levels of ability. I look at all of us and marvel at how far we've managed to outdistance the MonSter in this area. Maybe It would prefer that we sit around and do nothing but cater to Its whims: sleep, eat, brood over losses, let our minds and bodies turn to mush. This is one area where we haven't given in to Its demands. I can't remember the last time anybody in our group even hinted at being bored. Most of us can now join Tara in greeting each morning with enthusiasm and wonder.

When we began to talk about our sideline (or mainline!) activities, virtually all of the ladies contributed in great detail to the discussion. But, instead of turning this chapter into an arts-and-crafts, gardening, or pet-care instructional manual (maybe that's an idea for later?), we'll concentrate here on how having MS led us to those interests or allowed us to pursue them. We'll also include some of the tips and gimmicks we've come up with to get past the physical limitations we encounter in our hobbies. We do this in the hope that others, no matter what level of apparent disability they've reached, will find viable ideas for turning empty hours into fulfilling, fun, constructive times.

Dee I really enjoy writing and have always done so. Before I had MS, I didn't have time to be serious about it. I am now seriously studying writing and am writing almost every day. It's something I plan never to give up now.

Of course, writing is the first of my interests that I'd have to mention, too. Putting together *Women Living with Multiple Sclerosis*, then actually having it accepted by Hunter House for publication, offered me my first spark of hope that MS didn't have to mean the end of my writing dreams.

When I first gave up my job at the newspaper and stopped taking freelance work, I was at a loss. I didn't have an editor standing beside me to give me story assignments or set deadlines for when they had to be completed. I wanted to write, especially after the idea for *Women Living with Multiple Sclerosis* came along and the Flutterbuds agreed to join me in its creation. But my head contained only a jumble of thoughts that were too disorganized to ever make their way onto paper.

I was tired all the time, so much so that when I tried to write, my mind backed way from the boggling specter of all those empty pages that needed to be filled. I kept trying, mostly because I'd made a commitment to the Froup, and they cheered me on. Little by little, I learned to make adjustments in my modus operandi. I learned to write when I had the best control of my thoughts, usually early in the morning. I learned not to even try to put words together when I was tired; I'd only end up so frustrated I'd have to quit and would dread returning to the task for fear that there'd be a repeat performance (or nonperformance). When my fingers got too numb to find the right keys on the computer, I resorted to a voice-recognition program to do the typing for me. I saved almost every word of the Froup's conversations that I thought could possibly be useful in a book and catalogued the files with enough detail to let me easily find what I wanted. The system worked! After exactly a year, the Flutterbuds and I had reached our goal!

That success, the completion of *Women Living with Multiple Sclerosis*, was my first proof that I could get around the limitations that the MonSter wanted to impose on me, my writing, and most of my other interests. I found that persistence, along with trial and error, frequent revamping of techniques, and a dose of self-coddling when the occasion called for it was the key. I still follow the protocol I set up for myself during that time. I write when I'm rested and alert and let it go when I know that trying would be an exercise in futility. I use a mild form of self-discipline; I make myself stick to it for just an hour or two at a time, then move on to something entirely different, and apply the same success tools to whatever that "something" happens to be.

But don't you hate when writers write on and on about writing? On to something else....

Nadiza I have taken some sewing classes and quite recently developed a real passion for sewing. I'm slow, though. Even when I took the classes about seven years ago, I was much slower than the rest of the class. My fingers are often quite stiff and don't have the range of motion that they used to. That, coupled with loss of feeling in my fingers, has slowed me down. I have found some pins with large glass balls at the end that have made things a bit easier for me.

Robin Those pins with the balls on them are lifesavers! Also, it helps if you have a basket or special cabinet to keep all your supplies in one place (threads, scissors, tapes, pins, glues, etc; there are a lot!), so you don't have to keep getting up and down.

Me That really does help, Robin. When we remodeled last year, I moved an old china cabinet up from the basement and put it in our new "all-purpose" (office/television/sewing) room. That's where I keep my sewing stuff now. It's much easier to have everything in one place, especially since most of my sewing supplies used to be in the basement. Now, I only keep patterns and fabric stored down there; I can make one trip at the beginning of a project, and that's all the running (ha!) up and down for the duration.

Sewing is one of my greatest pleasures, discovered long before I found out I had MS and rekindled once I had the time and the initiative to overcome the little problems involved. My sister Joyce taught me to sew when I was seven years old, and my mother left me a legacy of tricks and tips that have honed my sewing skills. But there have been times when I wasn't exactly thrilled that the MonSter insists on sitting with me at the sewing machine. I've had to rethink some of Mom's hints and adapt them to accommodate Its presence.

I put my cutting board (two of them, if I'm working on something big) on the floor now and scoot on my rear to access the correct angles to position the scissors. I store my pins (long t-shaped ones from my mother-in-law's drapery business) on a big magnet instead of a pincushion, which lessens the chances that most of them will end up on the floor. I do almost the whole construction by machine now, including hems that I used to insist on doing by hand. When Mom died, I inherited her serger (Mom to the rescue again!), which makes all the finishing work less of a hassle for uncooperative fingers—no need to press under those teeny-tiny raw edges anymore!

Nadiza   I failed the sewing classes I took when I was in school. But I don't let a little thing like a failing grade hold me back! I've kept on sewing, and I keep finding ways to get around the problems I encounter. My fingers get very stiff at times, and I had trouble replacing the fragile pattern pieces in the their original envelopes. So I got some big clasp envelopes to put the patterns in. I cut the fronts off the original pattern envelopes, then I stick them with clear packing tape to the outsides of the clasp envelopes to identify them. It's much easier for me to insert the pattern pieces in the new envelopes without the worry of tearing them.

Me   I'll give you an "A" for that idea, Nadiza. I do something similar. I use gallon-sized plastic zip bags, stick the pattern envelope inside so it shows through, and then fold the pattern pieces (no need to worry about following those pesky, precise fold lines to make them fit!) and enclose them.

Margo Roy adapted my sewing table to a higher level, so I don't have to lean over so far to cut things out. It's been a lifesaver. Those pins that y'all have been talking about that are extra long and have the big heads are a wonder, as is my rotary cutter. I'm less likely to go for the more difficult patterns that I used to do, but that's okay with me. There are many cute, popular styles that are very simple to put together, even with hands that don't work well.

Me I've managed to get past many of the physical obstacles when I sew, but I've found that my biggest challenge has been my cognitive mix-ups (besides the one that made me need four years to memorize how to thread my serger!). I've learned to buy only certain brands of patterns; some others contain directions that, to my mind, seem to be written in any language but American English. I take it for granted now that, even as I follow a simple pattern, at least once during every sewing session I'll put something together upside-down, inside out, or backwards. No matter how carefully I think I've figured it out, the fabric takes on a life of its own and repositions itself as soon as I look away. Knowing that it's going to happen reduces my chagrin when it does. I keep three seam-rippers on hand, so there's always one within easy reach. And I use them!

I almost never close my sewing machine and put it away now. When the urge (or necessity) to sew strikes, I'd probably decide it's too much trouble to haul it out again. So it sits in a place of honor in my office, on a drop-leaf table that I can leave closed for small jobs and then open to hold bigger pieces that would otherwise drag on the floor.

I've found that sewing provides a good break from any

other chore or hobby I might have assigned to myself. I can go to my sewing machine, let my years of experience kick in to dictate the rules, and let my mind refresh itself while my fingers (and the seam ripper!) and the foot pedal do the work.

Sewing has replaced reading as my great escape. Sometimes I read a book, and a day later I don't remember anything about it. At least when I sew, the finished product is there to remind me that I really did it. Too often I find a book on my shelf and can't remember if I've ever seen it before.

Helen I learned to read when I was three and haven't had a book out of my hand since. I buy them at yard sales, thrift stores, regular stores. I can forget about me when I'm reading about somebody else.

Tara I also do a lot of reading. Since I don't think I'd be able to go back to school to get my Ph.D., I educate myself! I order books on every subject that I am interested in. Each subject seems to lead to another one that I am just as interested in.

Nadiza Reading is a hobby of mine, too. I have tons of books on nature and how to identify birds, insects, flowers, trees, etc. I like to learn about the heavens and what makes the earth tick. I like mysteries, too, but I guess my great passion is how-to books on almost every subject. Sometimes I have trouble remembering what I've just read. But I don't let that stop me. I'll read it five times rather than give up.

Tara One thing I have to watch is that I don't work too much on any one hobby for a long time. I try to do something that requires fine motor skills and then switch to using gross motor skills. Then I might just do some reading or journaling. I also keep scrapbooks with cuttings from magazines that are related to arts or crafts. I cut out particular paintings or drawings that I can refer to when I am having trouble with a work-in-progress.

Ramia Scrapbooking is my passion. I got rid of the living room furniture (John did the physical stuff) and moved my big table in front of the window in there. On mornings when I don't have appointments or other special plans, I work on my scrapbooks. I just gave my folks an album commemorating their forty-fifth wedding anniversary, the family trip to Alaska, and Dad's seventieth birthday. It makes me feel good, because they really loved it and are proud of my work. I think it helps them put aside the MS and the realization of what I can't do anymore. It gives me a purpose and makes me realize I still have a lot to do and I'm still able to do it!

Dev One of my hobbies is drawing. I just got a drafting table a couple of days ago, so I can sit up straight and draw instead of having to hunch over at the table. It's much easier on my back that way. I also do a lot of drawing on the computer and make greeting cards and invitations for family parties. It's just too much on my legs to stand in a store and find the right card. I like it because I can make the card to match the recipient's personality, and I can write my own sentiment. I have some great printing CDs, too. So when I'm too tired or my hands don't work quite right, I use them. I like oil painting but have an awful time with colors because of my eyesight. So, I go back to using my computer to "paint."

Bunny When my first symptoms showed up, I started to lose some of the use of my hands. I was interested in making ceramics but didn't know if I'd be able to handle all the steps involved. I happened to find Plaster Crafts® one day at the store. They're like ceramics, but without the need to be fired; you just paint and glaze them. My first piece was not as good as I had hoped it would be, since my hands were very shaky, but I kept at it. I enjoyed doing it, and it seemed like therapy for my hands. When I was finished, I had accomplished something besides sitting on my butt all day. Painting these plaster pieces led to other crafts and crafting ideas. At the time, we were in financial straits and making crafts was my salvation for Christmas. That year everyone got a handmade gift. It not only made me feel better but made Christmas affordable for us.

I've put tape around some of my brushes to help me hold them better. Paul has given me his magnifying visor that he uses for jewelry repair, so that I can see the fine details that need to be painted.

If I hadn't had to quit working, I wouldn't have discovered this hidden talent. Paul tells me I should start a business with my crafts, but that's something to think about later. In the meantime, I can do them just for the enjoyment they give me. They make me feel that I'm worth something again. I'm able to laugh at whatever hinders me from doing all that I used to do, because I've found new things to do instead!

Dee   That is so neat to hear, Bunny. I'm the same way—not very crafty. At least I wasn't until I discovered those little plaster pieces, too. I found children's banks and painted them—one for each grandchild. It's fun to hear that we started our crafts projects the same way and that they do so much for our self-esteem.

Nadiza   I used to love making pottery. When I started having problems with numbness and fatigue in my hands and arms, I had to put the dreams of a potter's wheel behind me. I didn't let it get me down, though. I went back to making ceramics instead. I can't draw freehand. Okay, I can draw freehand, but it's like my singing—bad! But I found that if I have something with form to work with, like a ceramic piece, I'm really quite good. I did find that I had to make adjustments with ceramics, too. If my hands were shaky and I wanted a piece off the shelf, I would ask someone to carry it to my work area. I would rather ask for help than give up on something I love so much. With or without MS, ceramics was the best thing that could have happened to me. I found out I had hidden artistic talent, and that did a lot for my self-esteem.

Tara   I have a new toy to use while drawing. It is a device that holds my arm up so that I don't have to work with those muscles that get tired so easily.

Robin   Someday I want to pick up my art/painting/drawing again. I imagine I'd want to find some gizmo like the Dr. Grip® pen. It's easy and comfy to hold; it doesn't get lost in my grip, even though I don't feel much in my right thumb and forefinger.

Dev   Those sound good, Robin. I'll definitely look for them. I still do some freehand drawing, but when my hands stiffen up, I have to quit what I'm doing and finish it later. I'm always looking for things that will make drawing a fun project instead of a chore. I like to use colored pencils, but now I have to get the fatter ones. I can't hold skinny pencils well anymore.

Kathey   That goes along with my theory—skinny is no good. But call the pencils "fluffy" instead of "fat," okay? They're sensitive.

Have you ever seen florist's tape? It's kind of soft and rubbery, with a nonslip surface. Maybe this could be wrapped around pencils, pens, and knitting needles to make them easier to hold.

Dev   That's what I need! I've had pencils go flying everywhere. Fluffy pencils? I kind of like that.

Me   Mom loved to crochet but had arthritis in her hands. I remember that one time she covered the handle of one of her big crochet hooks with foam and held it in place with soft fabric tape. She said it helped her to hold onto the hook. Maybe you could rig up something like that for your brushes?

Robin You know, I think you can buy some kind of gizmo like that. It is a rubber thing for people with arthritis that can be slipped onto pencils. Something like that could work for anyone with problems holding brushes. Thanks for the idea, JL and Kathey!

We have some Froup members who spend their leisure time hunting down collectibles.

Margo I collect teacups and have a small doll collection (I mean the collection is small, not necessarily the dolls). The teacups started years back and have developed a history of their own. I love each and every one, even when I have to take them all down and wash them. And yes, I use them from time to time. That's my way to make myself relax. I put flavored coffee in them, create my own "international moments." I take my special cup of coffee and then go curl up with a good book and my blankey.

Dee I collect teacups, too! I like to drink out of them when I have friends over. It seems so special to drink out of pretty cups, especially early in the morning. It puts me in the right frame of mind for the day.

Vicki That's why I like drinking my coffee out of my Looney Toons® cup every morning. That puts me in the right frame of mind for the day.

Laura I collect Barbies®. I started by replacing some of my childhood dolls that I'd given away. I now have lots of beautiful dolls. To me, they are like art. The childhood ones bring back memories, fond or bad ones, but all part of the crazy quilt of Laura.

I also help run science fiction conventions, collect original pieces of science fiction art, read, read, sew, and bead. I also like to cook, when I can do it right.

Helen I spend a lot of time video gaming. That sounds like an odd hobby for someone my age, but I am finding that there is an entire "subculture" of adult gamers, most of us thinking we are each the only one around. I find that playing just about anything on the computer keeps my fingers and my mind nimble.

Me That's true, Helen. At least that's what I tell Ron when he notes that I'm playing solitaire again.

Helen I also got interested in genealogy about five years ago, when I realized that there are no complete records of either side of my family. It's like trying to put together a very elaborate puzzle with all the pieces turned over and several missing. That, too, makes me think and keeps me busy. Maybe once every six months, I find a clue and off I go again, tracking down another elusive ancestor. If I can, I do the tracking in person. If not, I do it on the computer.

Kim My genealogy research is coming along great! I discovered that Keith Carradine is my cousin (okay, somewhat removed). I wrote to him for information on the family tree. At the same time, I asked him if he would like to do something for the MS cause. I wonder if I'll ever hear from him....

Kathey I guess my only real hobby is travel. I love to take day trips and have learned to schedule them so I'm relaxed and can take my time and rest as I need to.

I have travel books from nearly every state and a lot of foreign countries. That's how I plan my trips. I get brochures about the area and see what there is to do and how accessible the places are that I want to visit, and then I plan it all out.

Kim I just sent for a whole package of brochures from Arizona. I used to love to travel; now I collect picture books and look through them instead. It's not the same, but I can at least take a mind journey to any place, even the places I wouldn't be able to go to if I didn't have MS. Before I discovered this, I was so limited. Now the world is my trip!

Nadiza My most recent accomplishment is learning to play the piano. It's difficult on some days because of stiffness and loss of feeling in my fingers. The memory problem pops up also. I can be playing quite happily, and then I hit a brain fog and can't remember what note I'm looking at. Sometimes I tell my brain to move one finger, but another moves instead.

I see all these obstacles as challenges. I find ways to go around them rather than let them stop me dead in my tracks. If I see that some project would be too complicated for the limitations that MS has put on me, I just do something simpler that is within my capabilities. A compromise is better than giving up.

Bren My biggest hobby is being right here online. I love being on the computer, and the MonSter has yet to take away my typing (or my sense of humor). [We'll vouch for that!]

If not for the MonSter, I wouldn't be hosting support chat sessions for folks with MS. I would have never met the wonderful groups of folks that come into my chats. I definitely "put one over" on the MonSter by hosting these chats. When I get to talk to someone that is newly diagnosed and can help with his or her fears, *man!* that just thrills me. It makes me feel like I'm making a difference in the MS community. It gives me a great feeling of personal accomplishment, especially when that newly diagnosed person says "Wow! I feel so much better knowing I'm not alone in all this and knowing I don't have to be so scared." [Bren is also the contributing editor for a monthly MS e-mail newsletter. Folks who'd like to contact her may do so at hostahthbren@aol.com for information on her chats and the newsletter.]

Kim I think my computer is the thing that keeps me from going nutso. I've designed my own website and would like to get into helping other people design theirs. Then there is my genealogy research and answering e-mails from the Froup. I do have a very short attention span. I find that I can go back and forth to the mail or research and rejuvenate my mind in between by playing games or something.

Jamie I like to play Scrabble®. [I'll vouch for that! Jamie and I spent nine days together a couple of years ago, much of it over a Scrabble board. Jamie can't see much and can't move her hands well, but she can make a word out of any seven letters. She beat me every time!] I also listen to music and collect salt-and-pepper shakers and Harley-Davidson memorabilia. I ride a Harley when I feel well enough. Nobody will let me drive one now—could it be because I am blind in one eye and can barely see out of the other? I like to write poetry when I can see well enough. I like to joke and talk online with my Flutterbud sisters; they have saved my life on more than one occasion.

Nadiza I felt like a no-talent imbecile when I was growing up, so the ability to do anything now with any measure of success has given me a great deal of pleasure. I've learned to do new things all along, from baking my own bread to canning my own foods. There is just this great feeling of being special because I did it myself. To me, the world is still full of magic. Being able to do something new makes me one of the magicians.

Margo I spend a lot of time now visiting with my kids and grandkids. That and keeping in touch with the sister-friends I've found online make me feel that I haven't dropped off the edge of the planet. I still feel like a real person with a real life, instead of the shadow some of my ex-coworkers seem to think I am.

Dee But that, too, is a gift, Margo. In fact, it is one of the greatest gifts: being able to spend quality time with family, aging parents, children, grandchildren, friends. Al and I also get to spend a lot of time together. Most of that is good!

Helen Then I have my pets.

There we have the perfect opening line, from the perfect person to start the discussion on this topic. When we started to talk about hobbies, nearly all the ladies mentioned their pets as one of their time-enriching, sanity-saving pastimes. It appears, though, that caring for and interacting with pets is more than a hobby for our ladies—it's a passion! We've had many discussions about our animal companions, enough, again, to fill a book in itself. For now, we'll look briefly at how our pets make our lives with the MonSter more bearable (no pun intended—none of us has a bear in the house!). We also give a few tips on choosing and caring for pets when the MonSter wants to put a limit even on that.

Back to Helen, who is probably the Froup's "leader of the pack" when it comes to kinship with animals:

Helen Janni and I have an eccentric number of pets, mostly unplanned, but all very welcome and loved. We currently have six dogs and two cats in a city where three pets is the limit without a fancier's permit and five is the limit with a permit (shhhh!).

Helen is usually the first person we turn to for advice about pet care. Most of her animals were orphaned (she hand-raised them from birth), abused, or handicapped when she got them. She has nursed all back to health and happiness and is even training Chance to be a therapy dog, to visit folks who are homebound, sick, and lonely.

Helen I've always had dogs, but they were mostly medium- to large-sized ones. Now, with the changes in my physical condition and energy level, my tiny dogs are just right. I can carry T'Belle and Chance up the stairs, pick them up and put them into the tub, or do whatever needs to be done. My little dogs came into my life at just the right time.

Joy I used to train my bigger dogs to jump into and out of the tub for baths. Now, I'm not sure I could keep up with grooming a big dog. For me and my symptoms, small dogs are the best choice.

Robin I have a boxer. She's big but requires almost no grooming. There are times when I lose my balance; she is right there for me to lean on, sweet thing that she is!

Me We have a medium-sized dog and a small one. They're both hairy and need lots of grooming attention. They also like exercise, and I honestly believe that they are the reason I'm not in a wheelchair all the time. Sometimes I've *made* my legs work, for the sake of the dogs.

These guys are both getting old; I know I'm beyond the point where I can train and otherwise keep up with a new puppy. So Ron and I plan that, when our dogs leave us, we'll adopt a couple of rescued greyhounds. I understand that they're well trained when they arrive. And, they're so relieved to get away from the tortures of the race that they settle down to being very affectionate, contented couch potatoes. That's my idea of the perfect canine companion for an MSer.

Nadiza Eleven years ago, I ran into a real pet problem. I was newly diagnosed with MS, and I had a brand-new baby. I had two dogs and a cat that needed to go to a vet. There was no way I could handle even one dog with a babe in my arms. The solution came in the form of a vet that makes house calls. She has a kind of motor home, outfitted with veterinary equipment. It's wonderful because the animals all get taken care of at the same time.

Kathey We have one of those here. In fact, it's the vet I use. The prices for the services are the same as they are in the office. It's very convenient.

Then there's the "Bark and Wash." You can take your pets there and have them washed and dried. Or, for half the cost, they supply shampoo, towels, and a blowdryer, and you do it yourself. All the sinks are at chest level, with one lower tub in case you want to sit to bathe the pets. Very accessible!

Kathey's interests and affection extend to more than the usual dogs and cats. She has a cat, a parrot, two cockatiels, a rat, a dwarf bunny, and a white rabbit (Elmo, the dog, died recently).

Kathey They give me love when I need it, something to keep me busy when I don't have energy for more tiring pursuits. It's comforting to have a dog or cat on your lap, some little creature to cuddle with, who doesn't ask what's wrong, just knows that something is wrong and wants to help.

Chris I just have one dog, Bitsy. She keeps me company all

day when I am alone. I would be lost without her!!! She even sleeps with us at night!!!

Debby My toy red poodle Muffin can sense when the MonSter is about to rear its ugly head. She sticks right by my side for a couple of days before I have an exacerbation. While I am sick, she will not leave my side, even to eat.

Kim I've been thinking about pets and how they change us and change with us. I'd been trying to play with Hannah. One of our favorite things is to jog down the hall with her running behind me, holding a rope between us. Then we turn around and I tell her to take me back, and she runs me back to the living room. After falling on my face, it dawned on me that this isn't really doable anymore. We have had to adapt to that. Steve is there for her rough-and-tumble play. I've settled for just sitting on the floor and roughing it with her!

Joy Oh, doggies love for us to get down on the floor with them! We aren't showing dominance that way, so they're more comfy and relaxed.

Sally I have cut back from the number of pets I used to have. I want to be able to devote enough time to each of them. Now I have Sandy, my golden lab helper dog that I trained myself. This gal sticks by my side all the time. She automatically picks up things I drop, besides getting the things I ask her to get. She understands most words, but I sometimes use a laser pointer to let her know what I need her to get. Outside, she pulls my wheelchair and I steer by using the leash, which is hooked onto the handle of my chair, as a tiller. She loves to pull. Once I got stopped by a cop for going twenty-six miles-per-hour in a fifteen miles-per-hour zone. He didn't ticket me; he just stopped to let me know how fast Sandy was going and to meet her. I think this dog is closer to me than any other being has ever been.

Sally, even at her cutback level, still has her share of "other beings." In addition to Sandy, she has a miniature saltwater reef aquarium, with scores of fish and other water creatures whose names I'd never heard before. Clams, sponges, a dragon gobi, and a "big old snail" also live there. To top it off, she has an albino kingsnake that she rescued.

Then there's Joy, who has four dogs, one cat, and several well-stocked aquariums. Some of our ladies say that if they can choose what to be in the next life, they'll come back as one of Joy's animals.

But I think they'd be happy assuming a life with any of the Flutterbuds. If the numbers are any indication, the ladies in our group are super-committed to life in every form. I've seen about forty dogs, twenty cats, and an assortment of birds, fish and other creatures pop up in our conversations.

That doesn't even take into account the "wild" creatures we've welcomed. Marge frequently tells us about her encounters with deer and a number of other creatures in her yard. Her fascination with hummingbirds inspired both Joy and me to set up feeders for them within sight of our houses. (There's a perfect pastime for a heat-intolerant MSer—the hummers are most active on summer evenings, so we can actually leave our air-conditioned houses to sit outside and watch them without rousing the MonSter!). Sally likes hummingbirds, too; she has a special red hat that she wears when she wants to attract them to her apartment balcony.

I've wondered if the stronger-than-usual connection between the ladies in the Froup and their pets (and let's not forget all the plants we keep) is more than just a way to fill our time. Could it spring in some fundamental way from our need to escape from that other nonhuman creature we're connected with? I think that surrounding ourselves with living things, caring for them and letting them care for us, is a way that we can step outside our silly bodies and experience life through the lives of creatures that can never be bothered by the MonSter.

Helen Yup! They love us when we're stumbling around, when we have brain farts, when we're too fatigued to pay attention to them. They just love us anyway. They don't understand that this condition isn't a "normal" way to be, so they take it in stride. When my bigger dogs were here, if I fell, they'd help me up. My little ones can't do that, of course, but they make me smile; they care for me and love me when I'm having a bad day. Sometimes, they just are there for me when I need to reach out and feel another living being.

Me I think that getting involved in "other" life helps us forget how stinky ours can be sometimes.

Nadiza That's true. Having something that depends on us helps to focus some of our attention away from ourselves. It makes us feel more "able."

Kathey And doesn't it help us to look at life from their point of view? How can I whine when I look at these animals? They take life for what it is, without complaining. All they want is some attention and love (okay, and food). All they ask is for me to love them. So, I do. And, I learn.

15
Living Beyond Our Limits

Kim   I have to tell you all something. I've held back on saying this for a while, because so many in the Froup are having a bad time. It's weird that I've worried about that, because it's great news! For the last three weeks, I have felt better than I had in a year and a half. I thank The Powers That Be for giving me this good time to catch up on having fun! Believe it or not, I can even pitch a decent softball now! I got a mitt the other day, and Steve and I have played catch several times. He says I have a really good arm. You know, I was never athletically inclined. Now I have MS, and, for the first time in my life, I learn that I can do something well physically. That made me just about the happiest person on earth! I love my life! All of you who feel bad, please take some of my joy and use it for yourselves!

This note from Kim reminded me of myself. Not that I could ever pitch a decent softball or any other kind of ball. I don't expect to find out that, because I have MS, I can. But, looking back over my own life since the MonSter became an active participant in it, I recalled many times that some personal accomplishment, some small triumph, made me, like Kim, "just about the happiest person on earth." My happiness and wonder was enhanced by the realization that my most memorable victories have been possible, not in spite of MS, but *because* of MS.

One of those "small achievements" was when I decided to paint my living room. I knew I wouldn't be able to stand on a ladder, hold a roller, paint a straight line with a brush, or see the places I missed. So I left the existing paint as a base coat, then dipped a scrunched-up plastic bag into different shades of the same color, and *splatted* it all over the walls. It was impossible to mess up, and I had a great time doing it. Ron and Karen and Julie almost had to restrain me from splatting the rest of the house while I was at it. Since then, I've seen lots of ads in home improvement magazines and paint stores, giving instructions and selling kits to do exactly what I did. I didn't need instructions or special kits—I just needed to find a way to get out of the Beast's chains to spruce up my living room.

There have been bigger, life-impacting victories, too. Having MS forced me out of the cocoon I'd held tight around myself for most of my life. I've always been kind of shy about speaking in front of people. I could manage to do a Scripture reading in church or read the minutes of a meeting, but only if I had a well-rehearsed text in front of me. The thought of standing in front of a roomful of people and talking about myself, then giving impromptu answers to spontaneous questions, sent me into paroxysms of fear. Since the publication of *Women Living with Multiple Sclerosis*, though, I've been asked to speak at MS support groups, MS Society dinners, several colleges and high schools, and in online conferences. Before each, I've told the MonSter and Its slow-witted, slur-tongued influences to go take a nap. Then I've asked the Lord to be in my mind and in my heart and on my lips (or my fingers, if I'm typing). Each presentation has been enthusiastically received, and I've met many inspirational people in the process.

Maybe, as I added up my recollections, I got a bit too enthusiastic or lost track of reality. When I told the Flutterbuds that I wanted to thank the MonSter, even *embrace* It, for the gifts It has

given me, some of them tried to put me back on a more cred-
ible track.

Joy I hear you, but I hate the term "embrace" when it comes
to the MonSter. I refuse to do that. I may have to accept MS,
but I will never welcome it. No matter what lessons it may
teach me, or what hidden joys I find in my life as an indirect
result of having MS, I will never love the MonSter. Given the
chance, I will kill It *dead* and smile as I do so! And I know
that you would, too, JL. There's a big difference, to me,
between embracing the lessons and/or the good things we
find as a result of having MS and embracing the MS itself.
Do you follow me?

Me I do, and I even agree with you, Joy, that there's a difference. But I can't deny that MS has brought me many gifts,
gifts that changed my life and let me live out my dreams. I
can't accept the gifts without welcoming the giver. It sounds
like an empty truism, I know, but it's reality for me. Maybe I'll
hate the MonSter and curse Its existence someday when I'm
confined to bed and covered with piss and shit and drool. I
can only pray that I'll find reason to embrace It even in that.

Kathey Speaking as a nurse who is used to cleaning up body
wastes, if it's your own crap you're covered with, that's easier
to deal with, huh? Or would that be harder? I guess it all
depends on your attitude. Personally, I'm giving myself till
the end of this month to hold onto the anger that I've had;
then it's positive thinking for this girl.

Obviously, for some reason, I need the "poor me,"
"madder-than-hell" attitude for now, because every time I
snap out of that, it comes back and bites me in my oh-so-
adorable butt.

Me You're right, Kathey, you *do* need your anger now. It's part of the process of acceptance. If you're angry, that means you're not in denial. You've already gone through that first step toward acceptance. You know that, though, don't you?

Kathey Yeppers, but I liked denial a *lot* better. I know I am "intellectualizing" my MS. That's the only way I can deal with It right now. I figure if I can take It apart, piece by piece (MouSepoopie by MouSepoopie, so to speak), I can figure It out. Or at least control It in some way, control the effect that It has on me. I fear It, almost constantly. It's not always fear of the same thing. It's an ongoing process: fear, learn, conquer, learn, fear, conquer, rejoice, learn.... So, do you pick It apart, fear the cognitive crap (or whichever is your worst MonSterbite), learn coping strategies, find treatments, whatever it takes to accept that little piece? And then, even then, is it *accepted?* Or does the equation just switch to 1+4=786 when it had been 1+4=33, because that makes it easier to take? Can you embrace the unpredictability? That's like trying to grab a handful of purple Gak [the slimy substance that Kat taught us to throw, figuratively or literally, at whatever aspect of the MonSter we wanted to smack, to express frustration, grief, and, sometimes, overwhelming happiness]—it slides away as soon as you think you might "have it."

What was my point? Oh, yeah, intellectualization—how the power of the mind can somehow negatively or positively affect the MonSter. Obviously, attitude is important. A positive one brings a different light to new or recurring symptoms. I've tried like hell to "will myself" into good days. I've also tried to allow myself bad days, you know, "just rest, just veg out, don't do a dang thing." The power of my mind isn't all it used to be.

Should I surrender? Nah. Give in? Possibly, to a point, in that acceptance involves admitting some sort of powerlessness. I can't control what this MonSter is taking from me, but

I can control how I react, how I take It into my life, and how I make that life mine instead of Its.

Joy Kathey, I think the intellectualizing you are doing is part of a natural process for many of us. Is trying to understand MS a way to assume control? Maybe, but for me, I think it is more just plain curiosity. If the MonSter were a physical entity, dead, lying in front of me, I'd probably still want to dissect It and find out what made It go.

Kathey I suppose that at some time we have to just accept that MS is part of our lives and embrace what It has been able to teach us about ourselves and about life in general.

Sharon There are times when I can accept, embrace, and thoroughly comprehend the blessings that MS has brought into my life (and not question that they could have come in a gentler, more pleasant way). That comes from knowing that embracing my demons keeps them from biting me in the ass. Then there are days when I am angry, and I can't find anything good about being the recipient of the MonSter's "gifts."

I have paid attention to the emotional roller coaster that comes with MS, and I've identified the cycles as the stages of grieving: denial, anger, bargaining, sadness, and acceptance. But with this disease, this is no closure to the grieving. With each loss comes another round—you have to start over each time.

I believe that, after having MS for many years, as you have, Judy, acceptance is effected by the realization that it's the emotional fight rather than the Beast Itself that wears you down. That's not to say that you do not empower yourself by seeking knowledge that will improve your quality of life or that you don't hope for a cure. I just think you have gained the wisdom, through experience, to find peace with MS.

Me Right now, my peace is tied into the wonder of looking back and being able to say, "Okay, that's why such-and-such happened." Everything bad that MS brought into my life, everything that seemed to be a drag or an annoyance or a pain or a real tragedy, has led to something new and wonderful. That experience has erased much fear from my life. It lets me feel real joy and hope instead, every time the MonSter grabs me. I hate to wear a Pollyanna face, and I wouldn't say any of this if it weren't real in my life. I know also that I can't take credit for a "positive attitude." I can only thank God that he stays close and holds my eyes open when I most need to see his presence.

Sharon   I agree, Judy. My fear has been replaced with faith that the Powers That Be want only the best for me. I have only to pay attention and accept the gifts. That might mean accepting some hardship and pain, but on the other side of that is a better me. I have to give up control and fear and believe the platitude, "this too shall pass and the best is yet to come." I can't do it all the time, but I'm getting better at it!

On a more corporeal level, we can also absorb and visualize our fear, to make it not an externalized "beast," but just part of who we are.

Joy   I don't want fear to be any part of who I am. I don't want MS to be part of who I am, either. The disease affects my body and, to some extent, my mind, but it cannot touch the true me. I am not my physical self.

Sharon   I don't believe you can separate yourself from fear by simply stating you don't want it to be part of you. At some point in our lives, we are all afraid. Fear is a normal, healthy emotion. It motivates us to seek protection from danger.

Nor do I believe I can separate myself, my soul, my entire being from the MS that I have. I don't want to. It is an integral part of some of my characteristics and beliefs. I might have achieved positive characteristics like compassion, tenderness, and vulnerability without the influence of MS.

But the fact remains that they came in as a result of having MS, so I have to welcome the package deal.

I've stopped viewing multiple sclerosis as an enemy and accepted It as a part of my life. I didn't end up crippled from the neck down because I came to that peaceful conclusion. That doesn't mean that I won't seek a cure or an improvement to my life, and my actions clearly show that.

I guess I am living with MS in a sort of symbiotic relationship. I don't want to fight anymore; I think the stress of fighting was dangerous to my health. The more I fought, through denial, intellectualization, and anger, the worse I got and the more scared and defeated I felt.

Joy   Different individuals react to MS and its symptoms in individual ways. The course of the disease, for me, has been milder than it has been for many of you, and I wasn't diagnosed until my late forties. My gratitude for all of those years that were virtually symptom-free has no doubt influenced my reactions since then. Like you, I've experienced grief, denial, anger, and fear, but my emotional transitions, like my symptoms, have been gentler and probably more temporary. I'm not saying that I refuse to allow an existing fear to be part of my life; it's just that fear, based on my experiences of MS so far, doesn't really exist for me at this moment.

Kathey   All we can do, it seems to me, is to deal with each new fear as it arises, on a day-to-day basis. Today, one of us might have a droopy face. Tomorrow, another might have blurry vision or something different to fear. But we made it through yesterday, didn't we? And we'll make it through anything that comes our way today or tomorrow.

Me   That's it, Kathey! I remember, back when I was first diagnosed, being so scared of all the different "disabilities" of MS that I read or heard about. Now, many years later, I've been through most of those things that I feared. I've been in a wheelchair (still am, sometimes), lost control of my bladder (still do, sometimes), had a droopy face and blurry vision (still have them, sometimes). But you're right—I've made it through all of that (still do, every time). I can look back and honestly say that nothing was as bad as I'd expected it would be. All of my fear was a waste of time and emotional energy.

Kim That's how I look at it. I can't face tomorrow until today, so I really don't fear what is going to happen later on. I just try to make the best of today, to be the best person that I can be for today. If that means embracing a MonSter, then so be it. Consider It embraced. I'm not making It my best friend or my soulmate. It's like my liver and lungs, just a part of me. I accept that It's there, but I don't worry about Its presence.

Joy We are each in our own canoe, drifting through life, with similar MonSters as stowaways. All I can say about my own unwelcome passenger is that its weight has slowed the boat's progress enough for me to enjoy the passing scenery, to identify my friends on the shoreline and wave at them, and to find time to muse about many things. Even those scary moments, when the Beast rocks the canoe and icy water splashes into my face, have a purpose. They wake me and make me more alert and responsive to my body, to my environment, and to others around me. Such are the "gifts" I welcome, the luggage that the MonSter brought along. Does this mean that I accept Its presence? Yes, in the sense that I accept the things I have no power to change, like rain on my face and storm clouds on the horizon. I have learned to go with the current—to not glance back over my shoulder too often and to anticipate breaks in the clouds.

Margo Is surrender the same as acceptance? No. Acceptance just means you've laid down weapons that have proven ineffective. You might not like what's happening, but you are no longer waging active warfare against something you cannot change. You find a way around the wall, over the wall, or under the wall, or you learn to go about your own life in the shadow of the wall.

Surrender means quitting. It's telling the wall that it has dominance over you.

Either way, it comes back to the same old adage. *Attitude is everything!* A positive attitude enables us to quit wasting energy on a force we cannot control and find other ways to deal with it.

Kim Acceptance: I can't walk today, so I'll use a cane.

Surrender: I can't walk today, so I ain't getting out of bed.

Margo There you have it, folks! Nine hundred and twelve pages of dialogue, distilled into two fabulous sentences! Thanks, Kim!

▲▲▲

Reading back over that discussion, I think we've stumbled upon another of the MonSter's gifts. It has trained us as semanticists and analysts! I'll take that gift, too, though. Hearing the other Buds' translations of terms like denial and fear and anger yanks me out of complacency. It adds new aspects to what I thought was a completed picture of my own relationship with the MonSter. It reminds me that, as Sharon said, there's no closure to the grieving process when you have MS. Today, I might sincerely "welcome" the MonSter. That doesn't guarantee that I'm immune to someday wanting to join Joy in her quest to track It down, kill It, pick It apart, and laugh the whole time. Maybe that's what Kathey means about needing fear and anger to keep that same fear and anger from biting her in her "oh so adorable butt." If we at least keep the possibility of those feelings in mind, it won't be such a shock when they show up.

And all of this round–and–round rationalization is leading me right back into another Pollyanna attack. The reminder that bleak days might lurk on the horizon is a blessing in itself. It encourages us to cherish the "Hug the MonSter" times even more.

Dee We have been given a huge gift. We have the time to touch the people in our lives, to take little children to parks, to talk with big children, to visit the lonely, to make a difference just by being there. We can take the time to make things that are lasting, to create things that are unique.

I know that Al and I wouldn't be able to spend this time together, if I didn't have MS. It would be hard, with the differences in our ages, because I'd still be working full-time. Now, it's as if I am retired too! Because of MS, we have precious time to use as we like. So, even though we have MS and all that it entails, we have the other side to balance it out. It's not so bad most of the time!

Bunny I'm like Dee. If I didn't have this condition, I'd still be working a full-time job and two part-time jobs, and I wouldn't have the quality time that I have now with my family. I wouldn't have discovered that I have a creative talent with my crafts and that I can share that with my stepdaughter. I wouldn't have realized what a wonderful husband I have; I'd be too busy working, working and working to pay attention to that. Having this illness, whatever it may be, has made me not only take time to smell the roses but also to appreciate their fragrance more.

Dev Mike and I used to have a rocky relationship, because we were always working. When we did find time together, all we did was argue about bills or about who needed to do what around the house. I also get to spend time now with my kids and grandkids. I have become a pet lover, and I know that is because of MS. I never had the time for animals before; now I have two cats and a dog, and I'm thinking about getting another dog. I've also been able to read more and learn more about the things that I was interested in but never had the time to find out about.

Dee's and Bunny's and Dev's (and other Buds'!) gratitude to the MonSter for time with their partners is high on my list, too. The ironic part of this is that for some time I resented, in many ways, the enforced all-the-time time I've had with Ron during these past years. I've had to rely on him to the point where I've wondered if there was anything left of me, or if I'd just incorporated myself into him. But, thanks to his unyielding commitment to making our life together easier, better, more fulfilled and fulfilling, I see that we have, in fact, incorporated ourselves into each other. He has enabled me to become more "me," which makes our "us" more "mine."

Kim After I was diagnosed, I thought all the worst things had happened to me. Mom died (the day after I was diagnosed). I lost some friends along the way. But the most wonderful things have happened to me, too. I found out that the friends that I lost were not true friends. I learned that true friends (like Rita) are there for me day and night, in sickness and in health. I learned that my work was just that. I can now look outside in the morning and not have to dread going to work. I can enjoy what I see now, with nothing to keep me from my enjoyment. I am living my own script. Nobody else is writing it for me now. Yes, I still have down days. I allow myself to have those. They make the good ones seem all the better. In many ways, MS has given me my life back!

Helen MS has given me time to think, to play, to relax, to be at ease with myself. I'm no longer constantly frantic about not having enough hours in the day to get everything done. There are times I wish I could be out there making money.

Then I remember that, if I was "out there," I might have a paycheck, but I wouldn't have time to enjoy it. I've learned to let go of my hubris and ask for help when I need it. When I came to the point where I had to have help, it ground my butt to ask. With some practice, though, it became easier. Now I don't feel that I have to get everything done by myself. That also gives me time. Time to enjoy life, even though it has changed. The best and biggest gift of all is having had the time to be here online and find myself a family of the heart!

Bren I have received many blessings along with my diagnosis of MS. I've realized that life is short, and we must live each day as if it were our last. I've seen that I needed to remove a lot of trash from my life, such as people who took me for granted or used me or lied to me. I have realized that time with my Al and my children is precious and should not be wasted. I have learned the value of honor and truth in my relations with people. I have learned to speak my mind, bluntly and honestly. I don't have energy for beating around the bush, nor for lying. I don't like it from others, so I don't do it to them. I've had to depend on God more, so my relationship with him has become stronger and much more personal.

Sharon Before I received and learned to accept the limitations that MS brought to me, I saw myself as huge and powerful. I could do all and be all to everybody through the sheer power of my will. I thought I had no needs. MS has taught me to ask for what I need or want, without feeling "less than." It has taught me to say, "I don't know," or "I can't." It has taken me much further into recovery [from addiction and child abuse] by teaching me that surrender and acceptance don't mean lying down and giving up. It has taught me the difference between "powerful" and "empowered." It has taught me the real meaning of love. I can't describe it; I just know it. I can feel it and see it in the eyes of my husband, my kids, and my friends.

Tara Having MS has given me the chance to say, "Enough! I can't do this anymore," and to alter my whole lifestyle. Without MS, I would not have had the courage to leave a successful career in special education and try my hand as an artist. In doing so, I have given myself a new life.

There's more! Because I have MS, I have met and fallen in love with my soulmate, Dean. Our local newspaper was running an article about my disability and my resultant career change. Dean is the photographer who came to my house to take a picture for the article. We (more than) hit it off immediately. He is all that I have ever wanted in a friend, companion, and lover. Together, we are weaving the fabric of our new, shared life. We are carefully selecting and keeping those threads that make up each of us and beginning to add those that describe what we have become together. The design of this fabric seems to be much richer than the sum of what each of us adds to it. We both watch in awe as that happens to us.

I am hungry for life now; before I felt I was clawing my way through it. I didn't see life, didn't see death, never learned the lessons in nature that are before me each day. I hadn't learned to absorb the details, to see the smaller things, to learn from everything that is around me. I hadn't learned to let life touch my heart and soul!

Robin I have come to appreciate my body more. When I look at other people, I want to tell them to not take their bodies for granted. This disease has forced me to slow down. I still work full-time, but I don't run at a breakneck speed anymore. I was always a do-it-myself type of person, sometimes a perfectionist, and I always wanted to do everything and get it all done. Now I've learned that it's okay to not get it all done, and it's okay to ask for help.

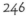

Ramia A couple of days ago, I needed to go shopping and knew I'd need help lifting and carrying everything I planned to buy. I am not good at asking for help from friends, but my next-door neighbor offered to take me. She went through the store with me, then unloaded everything to be checked out, and reloaded it in the cart after it was scanned. She told me to wait inside on a bench while she got the car; then she helped me into the car before she loaded all of my stuff into the trunk. After she got me home and made me comfortable, she brought everything into the house. She said that we'll do a shopping trip like that once a month from now on. I thanked her profusely, and she just said, "Please, let your friends help!" This made me realize just how valuable friends are. Because of MS, I have learned that I have some very good friends who feel hurt when I don't turn to them for help. Most people (friends *and* strangers) are happy to help, but it's up to us to let them.

Chris I have my own website now! That's something that I'm very proud of. If I didn't have MS, I'd be too busy working to do anything like that.

Kathey I'm a more compassionate person now, at work and in everyday life. I listen more, offer more compliments, help without being asked, touch people, and look them in the eye when I'm talking to them.

I've learned to not put anything off. I'm not dying, so that isn't what I have in mind. But maybe the next time I have a weekend off and the bald eagles are nesting near the lake, I might not be strong enough to go see them. So when I feel good enough to do something, I do it!

MS has taught me to express my emotions, negative and positive. To say, "I love you," or "I miss you." To say, "That hurt me," or, "I need you to be here with me," or even, "I

247

don't have enough room in my happy life for someone like you who makes me unhappy."

Maybe I've learned to express myself a little too much sometimes!

Debby I have found that I really do have the courage to fight the MonSter. I have learned to look for beauty in simple things, like being able to hold my little boy in my lap for a cuddle. I don't take things for granted like I used to.

Margo Because of MS, I am learning to be more honest. I no longer have the energy to be nice when I feel like speaking my mind to the contrary. I don't believe I've become a raging bitch, but I simply can't afford to "pussy-foot" around certain issues any longer. I speak more candidly, as my strength restricts me to saying what I mean more often than what people want to hear. I appreciate what I can do more than ever and am learning to let the rest go.

Sally Since I started having real problems with MS, I have learned new ways to do the things I want to do. I took up art and started making jewelry, the real kind, with gold and gemstones. I got a dog, and since I couldn't go through the strict training course at Canine Companions for Independence, I learned all I could about dogs and trained my own helper dog. I volunteer my time a lot to other folks with MS, folks who need help training their dogs, and folks who need help with Macintosh computers. In many ways the reward I get from helping others is so much more than the paycheck I used to get for working. I feel that volunteering is my way of earning the SSDI check that pays my rent. The best thing is that I can work when I'm able, as opposed to being on a schedule that I couldn't keep.

I've learned that laughter is the single most important tool we have to help us live with the MonSter. Laughing allows us to live with dignity when otherwise we might be too overwhelmed to cope with life at all. Laughter allows us to de-MonSter the strange things, the scary things, and the sometimes totally humiliating things that happen with MS. It helps us to not take every little blow to our egos as a catastrophe. The MonSter wants us to cry and be angry. We can take the wind out of Its sails by laughing in its face.

Jamie I can't see, can no longer drive an eighteen-wheeler, and have not worked since MS hit me. *But,* I have had a child, born two years after I was diagnosed and after being told I could never have one. Jaylon Starr is my miracle. Although she lived with me most of her life the hardest thing I have had to do is let my mother take over her care because of my physical limitations and my concern for her welfare and safety.

I consider MS a blessing. Because of MS, I have met the most wonderful people and learned more compassion for anyone who is suffering. I've learned to acknowledge God in all things. He has a plan for each of us, even though we might not understand it. I've learned to believe that he will provide what I *need,* not what I *want.* (If you want to hear God laugh, then just tell him what *your* plans are!)

Me I think that's true, Jamie, for all of us, whether or not we have MS!

Janis It has become clear to me that the Lord does not want me to be bitter about this disease. I have to remember that he allowed it in my life for a reason. Other people have told me that, because I have MS, I've influenced their lives in positive ways. If God can use me to touch people in some way, then that is what I will do.

I have that same assurance, Janis. That's where most of my gratitude for having MS arises. MS has made me alert to signs that God is directing everything I do and led me to the belief that whatever he uses as an instrument for his work, even a MonSter, can't be all bad.

Because I have MS, there have been occasions when I didn't have to search for proof that God was at work. The proof was right there, in my face, exactly when I needed it. This book is one absolute illustration of that.

Months ago, I approached the Flutterbuds about putting together a sequel to *Women Living with Multiple Sclerosis.* They agreed, and I began to work on it. At first, though, it seemed to go nowhere. We had a hard time focusing on my proposed theme of "living beyond our limits." Many of our ladies were going through rough periods that were impossible to acknowledge as blessings from the MonSter. That pushed me into an examination of conscience. I wondered about my motives for writing another book. Was I forcing the ladies into a frame of mind that wasn't authentic? Would the continued sharing of our experiences and ideas really be helpful to other MSers who might read them? What if we devoted however much time it would take to produce another book, and then discovered that no publisher wanted to take the chance that readers would want to accompany us again on the Froup's meanderings?

I wrote to the ladies and told them about my misgivings. I ended the letter with, "I guess it's time to toss the whole idea up to God, then wait for him to toss it back with instructions on what to do with it." They assured me that they wanted to go along with whatever answer I received. Less than forty-eight hours later, Jeanne, the acquisitions editor at Hunter House, called. She told me that Kiran (Rana, the publisher) wondered if we'd be interested in doing a sequel to *Women Living with Multiple Sclerosis.*

God knows it's sometimes hard for MonSter-muddled minds to hear and understand what is being said to us. Because I have MS, He spoke directly and clearly to let us know that he *wanted* us to write this book.

Nadiza Because I have MS, I have the chance to be part of a book that may help others deal with the disease. This makes me feel good. It makes me feel as though I am contributing to the world beyond my little circle. I want to let others know that adversity can be faced with dignity and a sense of humor. I wouldn't be able to say that without having experienced it myself.

Perhaps the greatest MonSter-gift that I've realized, not only in myself, but also in each of these ladies with whom I communicate every day, is the ability to be intensely in touch with our essential selves. We've learned to seek out the positive spiritual elements of our beings, nourish them, and enable them to take over where our flawed bodies fail us. MS has made us cultivate the one, most fundamental, component of our spirits that influences everything else about us. We've learned to hope. That allows us to focus on the upcoming day when researchers will announce that, finally, we can get up on our own feet and go anywhere we want to go. I think we'll go, first of all, to join Joy and our other fellow MSers. Maybe we'll embrace the (dead) MonSter one last time. Then we'll laugh.

The Beast Within
by Dev

What is this thing that lurks inside?
It steals my body and my mind,
It leaves me with a fear so strong,
I think and wonder, what is wrong?

I cannot walk the way I should,
I cannot run, I wish I could.
My eyes do not see like before,
I can't remember anymore.

What else will it steal in the morning light?
I cannot let it, I must fight.
How can I fight what I cannot see
This monstrous thing inside of me?

I must go on living and fighting this beast,
I will never give in, I must not cease.
Till one day I hear the words so clear,
Like an angel whispering in my ear:

Fear not this beast; it will go away.
There will be a cure one special day.
So I fight and I wait and I don't give in,
I wait patiently for this miracle to begin.

I'll run to a field spinning round and round,
A field of violets that surround.
I'll lift myself up and run through the trees,
With a smile on my face, I'm free, I'm free!

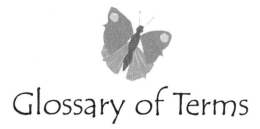

Glossary of Terms

adrenocorticotropic hormone (ACTH): hormone produced by the front pituitary gland. It controls the secretion of corticosteroids by the adrenal gland. In commercially produced form, ACTH is sometimes used to treat acute exacerbations of MS.

antihistamine: substance that reduces the body's response to a foreign substance (allergen).

autoimmune disease: disorder in which the body's defenses are turned against itself. Many researchers believe that autoimmune diseases occur when some agent, perhaps a viral infection or environmental contaminant, triggers the body's defense cells to destroy healthy tissue.

Baclofen®: a muscle relaxant used to treat spasticity in multiple sclerosis.

benign sensory MS: a type of multiple sclerosis which primarily causes impairment of sensory acuity; there is usually no loss of function of the affected area.

cardiac arrhythmia: an abnormal rate of contractions of the upper (atria) or lower (ventricles) chamber of the heart.

central nervous system (CNS): one of the main divisions of the nervous system of the body, consisting of the brain and the spinal cord. It is the chief control center for function and sensation in the entire body. An intricate network of nerves governs the workings of the body by carrying impulses or commands to and from the central nervous system.

Chiari malformation: bulging (herniation) of the brainstem and lower lobe of the brain (cerebellum) through the base of the skull into the spinal canal.

demyelination: destruction of the covering (myelin sheath) of a nerve.

Detrol®: drug used to control bladder spasms.

Ditropan®: drug (oxybutynin chloride) that relieves spasms. Commonly used to treat neurogenic bladder in MS.

evoked potential (EP), evoked response: tracing of brain waves, measured by placing electrodes on the surface of the head at various places, to record the length of time it takes for the brain to respond to specific stimuli.

exacerbation: recurrence of symptoms or an increase in the seriousness of symptoms of a disease or disorder.

fibromyalgia: painful condition affecting the musculoskeletal system, often identified by exaggerated pain reaction to touch at various trigger points on the neck, back, and torso. Frequently co-exists with MS.

immunosuppressant: agent used to reduce the ability of the immune system to respond to stimulation by antigens. Sometimes used as a treatment for multiple sclerosis, to prevent further autoimmune damage.

intramuscular injection: introduction of medication through a needle into a muscle.

lesions: spotty areas of destruction of myelin in the brain and spinal cord.

Lhermitte's sign: shock-like sensation radiating from the spine through the extremities, induced by flexing the neck or by sudden movements of the head. Common in many spinal cord injuries and disorders, it is often an early sign of multiple sclerosis.

magnetic resonance imaging (MRI): diagnostic procedure which uses radiofrequency radiation to view areas of the body in multiple planes. MRI of the brain and spinal cord is the most common method of diagnosis of multiple sclerosis. Spots of plaque (scarring) which appear on the brain and spinal cord are usually indicative of the presence of the disease.

myelin sheath: fatty covering of nerve fibers. The destruction of myelin in multiple sclerosis results in sclerotic (hardened) patches along nerve pathways, interrupting messages to and from the brain.

narcolepsy: disease characterized by sudden sleep attacks or sleep paralysis.

neurogenic bladder: urinary bladder disorder, often caused by diseases of the nervous system, which results in incontinence, urinary retention, or a combination of both.

optic neuritis: inflammation of the optic nerve, usually accompanied by severe eye pain and visual disturbances; frequently a first symptom of multiple sclerosis.

oxycodone hydrochloride: narcotic painkiller used to treat moderate to severe pain.

peripheral nervous system: the motor and sensory nerves outside of the brain and spinal cord.

periventricular region: area surrounding the four fluid-filled cavities within the brain. MS plaques are commonly found within this region.

placebo effect: beneficial result of drug treatment that occurs because of a patient's expectation that the therapy will help, even when the administered drug is composed of inactive substances.

plaques: hardened (sclerotic) areas of demyelination in the white matter of the central nervous system.

polypeptide: chain of amino acids, formed by partial breakdown of proteins or by connecting amino acids into chains.

prednisone: hormone (glucocorticoid) often used to treat inflammation and modify the body's immune response during acute exacerbations of MS.

primary progressive MS: type of MS characterized by progressive disease from the onset, with only ill-defined plateaus or remissions.

progressive/relapsing MS: type of MS characterized by disease progression from the beginning, but with clear attacks of worsening symptoms, with or without remission from those relapses along the way.

relapsing/remitting MS: type or stage of MS characterized by acute attacks with full or partial recovery and little or no disease progression between attacks.

remission: partial or complete absence of symptoms of an identified long-term disease. Remissions typically follow acute attacks of MS symptoms in the remitting/relapsing stage (or type) of the disease.

secondary progressive MS: type or stage of MS that often ensues after an initial relapsing/remitting course. The disease becomes more progressive, with possible continued occurrence of occasional relapse and less complete remission.

spinal tap (lumbar puncture): procedure in which the spinal column is punctured and cerebrospinal fluid withdrawn. Laboratory analysis of the fluid can reveal abnormalities that indicate the possible presence of MS.

subcutaneous injection: administration of medication by using a needle to place it in the tissue beneath the skin, usually on the upper arm, thigh, buttocks, or abdomen.

thalamus: one of a pair of organs that form most of the outer walls of the third ventricle of the brain and part of the back part of the front brain. It is part of the mechanism that produces complex reflex movements.

tremor: spastic movements caused by the uncontrolled tightening and relaxing of groups of muscles. Intention tremor, which occurs frequently in multiple sclerosis, occurs during conscious effort to use a limb for a particular function.

trigeminal neuralgia: painful inflammation of either of the largest pair of skull nerves. The trigeminal nerves connect to three areas in the brain and affect sensory and motor function in the face.

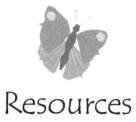

Resources

With the availability of the Internet, there's no need for any person with MS, or the loved ones of any person with MS, to be lost or alone in their daily battle with the MonSter. There are countless organizations, agencies, and individuals who can provide answers to questions about life with MS. This list is limited to just a few of the contacts we've found to be especially helpful. Most of them are, in themselves, databases of other potentially helpful connections. One Internet contact can connect to thousands of other resources for information, peer support, financial assistance, and just about any other need an MSer might have. Where possible, I've included snail-mail addresses and phone numbers in addition to web addresses.

NMSS: The National Multiple Sclerosis Society
... One thing people with MS can count on:
733 Third Ave.
New York NY 10017
(800) Fight-MS (344-4867)
www.nmss.org

Multiple Sclerosis Education Network
www.healthtalk.com./msen

Multiple Sclerosis Only!
www.msonly.com

Accordant Health Services
4900 Koger Blvd.
Greensboro NC 27407
(800) 948-2497
www.accordant.com
This organization is dedicated to management of chronic diseases; MS is one of their specialties. Their website features live forums, moderated chats, and many resources for information.

Rocky Mountain MS Center
701 E. Hampden, Suite 420
Englewood CO 80110
(303) 788-7667
www.mscenter.org
The Rocky Mountain MS Center is one of several facilities that accept donations of brain and spinal cord tissue for use in research at the death of an MS patient. Arrangements should be made well in advance. Necessary forms are available by contacting the center.

Doctors' Guide to the Internet
www.pslgroup.com/MS

Discovery Health (sponsored by Johns Hopkins Health)
www.discoveryhealth.com

Message Boards for MS on America Online
Type in AOL keyword "ah"
* Double click link for "Conditions A–Z" on the left side of the AllHealth home page
* Double click link for "Brain & Nerve Disorders"
* Double click link for MS message boards
* Follow prompts to get to other features, such as online chats. Most other servers provide similar areas.

WebMD

www.my.webmd.com

This site includes different forums for a wide variety of conditions. There are message boards and frequent live events (and archives of previous events). Go to the "conditions" prompt, find "multiple sclerosis," and then follow the prompts to whatever you're looking for.

People Helping People, Inc.

9250 Columbia Ave. D2

Munster IN 46321

(219) 836-2733

www.msphp.org

This organization was founded by our Nadiza's neurologist, Dr. Prasad, who also serves as its medical director. Its goal is to acquire living units or small homes where people with severe disabilities can live together and provide support to each other in a home environment. The organization hopes to expand what started as a local effort, to include the nation and, eventually, the world.

The Multiple Sclerosis Foundation

6350 N. Andrews Ave.

Fort Lauderdale FL 33309

(954) 776-6805

(800) 441-7055

www.msfacts.org/indexold1

At least two members of our Froup have personal websites that provide intimate glimpses into the lives of MSers, as well as medical information and lots of inspiration!

Kim has three attractive, helpful sites:
http://members.tripod.com/tink1960
and
http://home.earthlink.net/~tink1960
and
http://freepages.health.rootsweb.com/~tink/

Chris has a well-developed site, which she updates frequently:
Chris's "Happy Homeland"
http://members.aol.com/Chris12115/index.html

Invisible Disabilities Advocate (IDA)
www.invisibledisabilities.com
This is one of the most comprehensive personal sites I've seen. The creator of the site has MS and a number of other debilitating conditions. She tells a compelling story of her struggle and her ultimate triumph over catastrophe. She also shares the wealth of useful information she accumulated as she went about learning to live with disability. Whatever you need to know about MS or most other chronic conditions, you'll probably find it here.

For information on the ABC treatments for multiple sclerosis
Avonex
(617) 679-2000
www.biogen.com

Betaseron
(800) 788-1467
www.betaseron.com/index

Copaxone
(800) 887-8100
www.tevamarionpartners.com/mswatch

There are many excellent books about MS. Descriptions and ordering information can be found at:
www.wellnessbooks.com/ms/

The rest of the resources aren't necessarily directed at MSers, but can provide information about making the most of life with the MonSter:

The Association for Driver Rehabilitation Specialists
P.O. Box 49
Edgerton WI 53534
(608) 884-8833
(608) 884-4851, fax
e-mail: webmaster@driver-ed.org
www.driver-ed.org

The Driver Evaluation and Training Program for Individuals with Disabilities
Crotched Mountain Rehabilitation Center
One Verney Dr.
Greenfield NH 03047
(603) 547-3311
www.cmf.org
This is the base of Paul St. Pierre, who provided accessibility information for Chapter 11.

Links to manufacturers and distributors of assistive technology products for persons with disabilities:

www.abledata.com/Site_2/assistiv.htm

ADA Disability and Business Technical Assistance Centers (DBTACs)

These centers provide information, training, and technical assistance on the Americans with Disabilities Act. DBTACs can make referrals to local sources of expertise in reasonable accommodations.

(800) 949-4232

www.adata.org/dbtac

RESNA Technical Assistance Project

RESNA, the Rehabilitation Engineering and Assistive Technology Society of North America, provides information and referrals to help determine what devices may assist persons with disabilities and referrals to sources that provide assistance for purchasing, repairing, recycling, or exchanging assistive devices.

(703) 524-6686

(703) 524-6639, TTY

www.resna.org/hometa1

National Organization on Disability (NOD)

(800) 248-ABLE

910 Sixteenth St. N.W., Suite 600

Washington DC 20006

www.nod.org

Social Security Administration

(800) 234-5772

www.ssa.gov/SSA_Home

SSA Disability Information

www.ssa.gov/odhome

Medicare

(800) MEDICARE (633-4227)

The keyword "MEDICARE" on any World Wide Web browser

goes to an online home page that links to information about Medicare.

Americans with Disabilities Act
www.eeoc.gov/laws/ada

Toll-Free Numbers to Agencies
macdds.org

Index

H

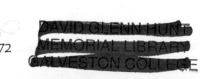

WOMEN LIVING WITH MULTIPLE SCLEROSIS
by Judith Lynn Nichols and her Online Group of MS Sisters.

In this book Judith Nichols and over 20 other women who formed an online support group share intimate accounts of their experiences with MS. Some stories are painful, some are funny, often they are both. The range of concerns includes family reactions; workplace issues and relationships; sexuality and spirituality; depression and physical pain; loss of bladder and bowel control. All topics are discussed freely and frankly, in the way closest friends do.

"The book is a validation of experience for those who have been in support groups, an invitation to those who have not yet done so, and a celebration of the wonder and pleasure that these particular women take in having found each other."
— Anne-Elizabeth Straub, CSW, *Inside MS*

288 pages ... Paperback $13.95

GET FIT WHILE YOU SIT: Easy Workouts from Your Chair
by Charlene Torkelson

Here is a total body workout that is perfect for office workers, travelers, and those with movement limitations or special conditions. The *One-Hour Chair Program* is a full-body, low-impact workout that includes light aerobics and exercises with or without weights. The *5-Day Short Program* features compact workouts for those short on time, and the *Ten-Minute Miracles* are a group of easy-to-do exercises perfect for anyone on the go.

160 pages ... 212 b/w photos ... Paperback $12.95 ... Hard Cover $22.95

COMPUTER AND WEB RESOURCES FOR PEOPLE WITH DISABILITIES *by* the Alliance for Technology Access

This book shows how people can use computer technology to enhance their lives. It describes conventional and assistive technologies, gives strategies for accessing Internet resources, and features charts relating access needs to software, hardware, and communication aids. Also included is a gold mine of Web resources, publications, support organizations, government programs, and technology vendors.

*384 pages ... 40 b/w photos ... 8 charts ... Third revised edition
Paperback $20.95 ... Spiral bound $27.95 ... ASCII disk $27.95*

MENOPAUSE WITHOUT MEDICINE
by Linda Ojeda, Ph.D. ... *New Fourth Edition*

Linda Ojeda broke new ground 15 years ago with this bestselling resource on menopause, giving women a clear understanding of menopausal changes and guidelines for effective self-care.

In this new edition she re-examines the hormone therapy debate; suggests natural remedies for depression, hot flashes, sexual changes, and skin and hair problems; and presents an illustrated basic exercise program. She also includes up-to-date information on natural sources of estrogen, including phytoestrogens, and how diet and personality affect mood swings.

352 pages ... 32 illus. ... 62 tables
Paperback $15.95... Hard cover $25.95

HER HEALTHY HEART: A Woman's Guide to Preventing and Reversing Heart Disease Naturally
by Linda Ojeda, Ph.D.

Heart disease is the #1 killer of American women ages 44 to 65, yet until now most of the research and attention has been given to men. This book fills this gap by addressing the unique aspects of heart disease in women and the natural ways to combat it. Dr. Ojeda explains how women can prevent heart disease whether they take hormone replacement therapy (HRT) or not. She provides detailed information on how to reduce the risk of heart disease through diet, physical activity, and stress management.

352 pages ... Paperback $14.95 ... Hard cover $24.95

MAKING LOVE BETTER THAN EVER: Reaching New Heights of Passion and Pleasure After 40
by Barbara Keesling, Ph.D.

With maturity comes the potential for a multi-faceted, soulful loving that draws from all we are to deepen our ties of intimacy and nurturing. Sex expert Barbara Keesling provides a series of exercises that demonstrate the power of touch to heighten sexual response and expand sexual potential; reduce anxiety and increase health and well-being; build self-esteem and improve body image; open the lines of communication; and promote playfulness, spontaneity, and a natural sense of joy.

208 pages ... 14 illus. ... Paperback $13.95

All prices subject to change

THE PLEASURE PRESCRIPTION: To Love, to Work, to Play — Life in the Balance *by* Paul Pearsall, Ph.D.

New York Times Bestseller!

This bestselling book is a prescription for stressed-out lives. Dr. Pearsall maintains that contentment, wellness, and long life can be found by devoting time to family, helping others, and slowing down to savor life's pleasures. Pearsall's unique approach draws from Polynesian wisdom and his own 25 years of psychological and medical research. For readers who want to discover a way of life that promotes healthy values and living, *The Pleasure Prescription* provides the answers.

288 pages ... Paperback $13.95 ... Hard cover $23.95

Just Announced!
PARTNERS IN PLEASURE *by* Paul Pearsall, Ph.D.

The much-awaited sequel to *The Pleasure Prescription* is coming in March 2001 — reserve your copy now.

WRITE YOUR OWN PLEASURE PRESCRIPTION: 60 Ways to Create Balance & Joy in Your Life *by* Paul Pearsall, Ph.D.

Dr. Pearsall offers this companion volume to *The Pleasure Prescription* for the many readers who have written asking for ways to translate the harmony of Oceanic life to their own lives. It is full of ideas for bringing the spirit of aloha — the ability to fully connect with oneself and with others — to everyday life. He encourages readers to disengage from the headlong rush and frenzy of Western life in order to feel the pleasure that comes from a calm acceptance of the world around us and the connection we have with others.

224 pages ... Paperback ... $12.95

WRITING FROM WITHIN: A Guide to Creativity and Your Life Story Writing *by* Bernard Selling

Writing from Within has attracted an enthusiastic following among those wishing to write oral histories, life narratives, or autobiographies. Bernard Selling shows new and veteran writers how to free up hidden images and thoughts, employ right-brain visualization, and use language as a way to capture feelings, people, and events. The result is at once a self-help writing workbook and an exciting journey of personal discovery and creation.

320 pages ... Third Edition ... Paperback ... $17.95

ORDER FORM

10% DISCOUNT on orders of $50 or more —
20% DISCOUNT on orders of $150 or more —
30% DISCOUNT on orders of $500 or more —
On cost of books for fully prepaid orders

NAME

ADDRESS

CITY/STATE   ZIP/POSTCODE

PHONE   COUNTRY (outside of U.S.)

TITLE	QTY	PRICE	TOTAL
Living Beyond Multiple Sclerosis... (paper)		@ $14.95	
Women Living with MS (paper)		@ $13.95	

Prices subject to change without notice

Please list other titles below:

		@ $	
		@ $	
		@ $	
		@ $	
		@ $	
		@ $	
		@ $	

Check here to receive our book catalog   ❑   free

Shipping Costs:
First book: $3.00 by book post ($4.50 by UPS, Priority Mail, or to ship outside the U.S.)
Each additional book: $1.00
For rush orders and bulk shipments call us at (800) 266-5592

TOTAL	_____
Less discount @____%	(_____)
TOTAL COST OF BOOKS	_____
Calif. residents add sales tax	_____
Shipping & handling	_____
TOTAL ENCLOSED	=========

Please pay in U.S. funds only

❑ Check ❑ Money Order ❑ Visa ❑ Mastercard ❑ Discover

Card #_____ Exp. date_____

Signature_____

Complete and mail to:
Hunter House Inc., Publishers
PO Box 2914, Alameda CA 94501-0914
Website: www.hunterhouse.com
Orders: (800) 266-5592 or email: ordering@hunterhouse.com
Phone (510) 865-5282 Fax (510) 865-4295

LMS- 9/2000